M000248858

beauty water

beauty water

everyday hydration recipes
for wellness and self-care

Tori Holmes

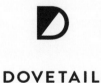

DOVETAIL

Copyright © 2019 by Tori Holmes

Photographs by Scott Gordon Bleicher, except for photographs on pages 22, 32, 42, 50, 60, 68, 80, 90, 100, 110, 120, and 151 by Britney Gill

Design by Lauren Brynn Lucas

Published by Dovetail Press in Brooklyn, New York, a division of Assembly Brands LLC.

All rights reserved. No part of this book may be reproduced, distributed, or transmitted in any form or by any means without the prior written permission of the publisher, except in the case of brief quotations used in critical reviews and certain other noncommercial uses permitted by copyright law.

Neither the publisher nor the author shall be liable for any complications, medical issues, or losses allegedly arising from any information in this book. You are advised to consult with your health-care professional with regard to matters relating to your health.

For details or ordering information, contact the publisher at the address below or email info@dovetail.press.

Dovetail Press
42 West Street #403
Brooklyn, NY 11222
www.dovetail.press

Library of Congress Cataloging-in-Publication data is on file with the publisher.

ISBN 978-1-7326952-0-7

First printing, April 2019

Printed in China

10 9 8 7 6 5 4 3 2 1

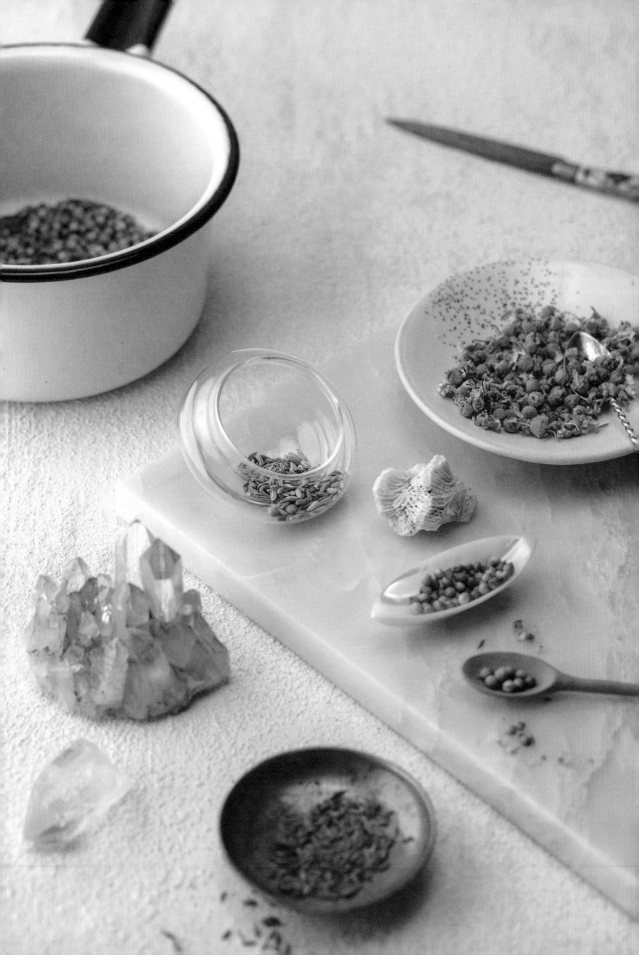

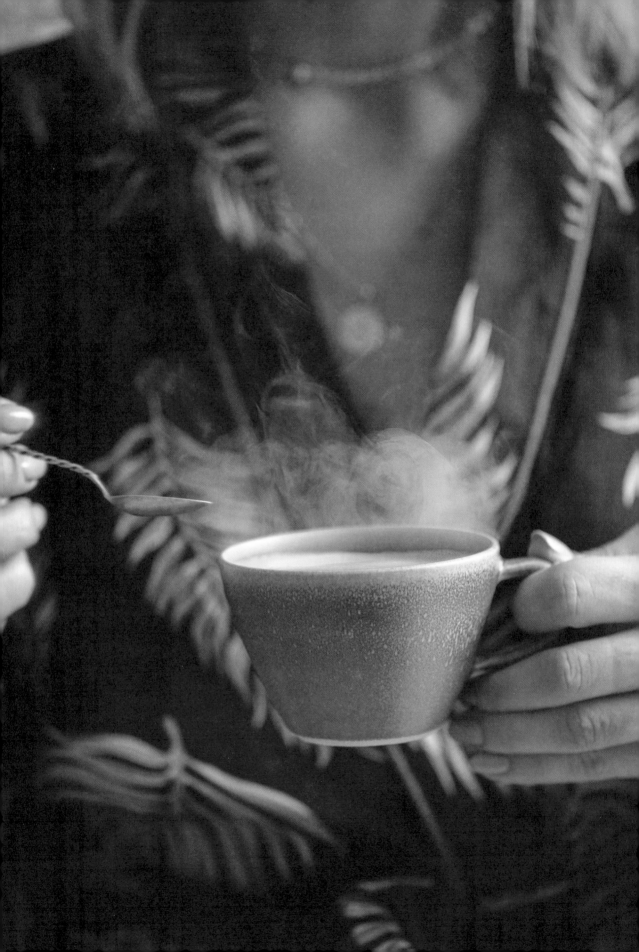

To my girls, Layla, Isalyn, and Olive—future women of
this world, I dedicate this book to you.
After witnessing your beautiful births, I cherish every
moment I am blessed to spend with you on your
journey to discovering the gift you offer to the world.

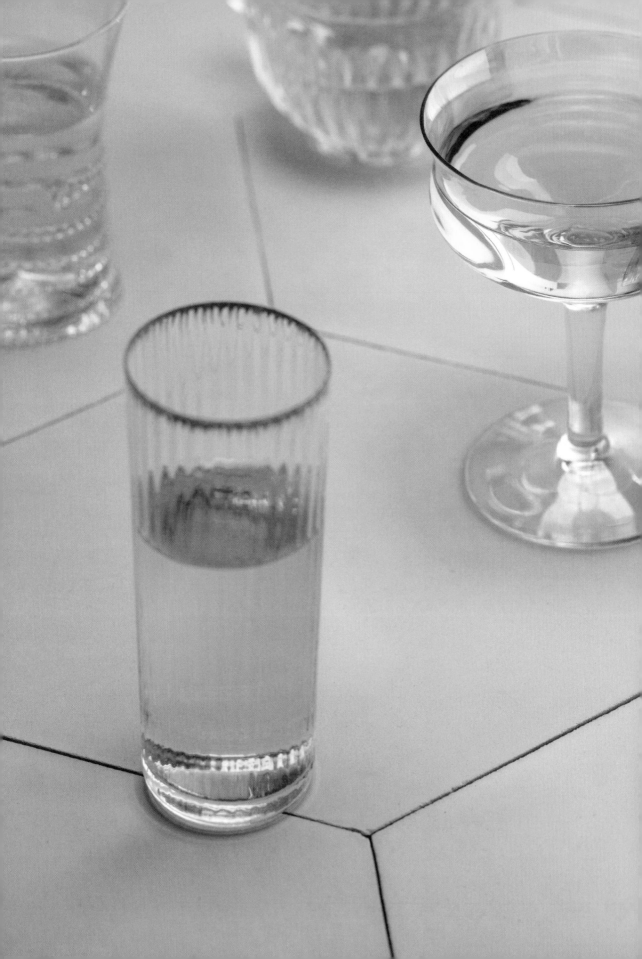

contents

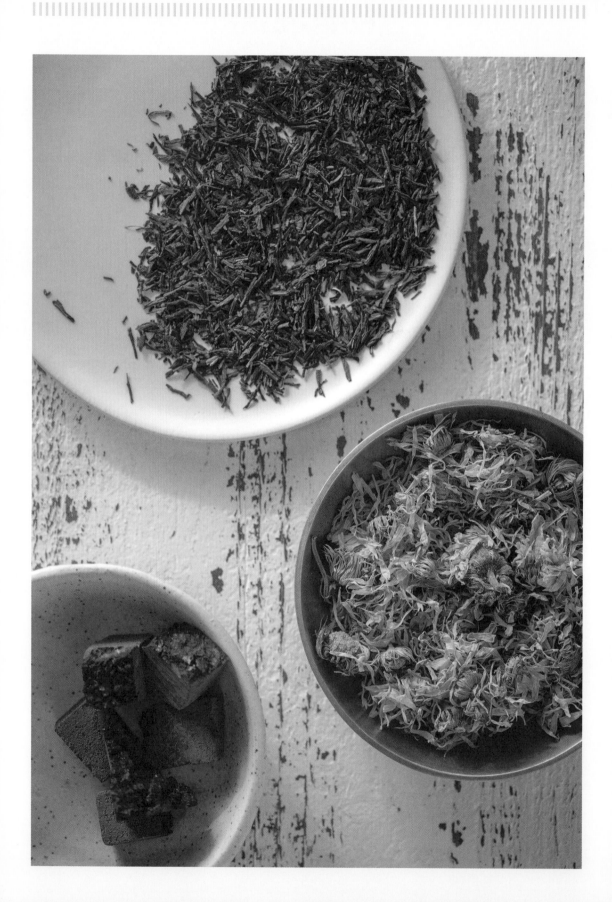

introduction

At the age of 21, I rowed across the Atlantic Ocean.

I embarked on this journey recognizing the row from the Canary Islands to Antigua as an extraordinary test of the human spirit. I knew it would be a life-altering experience, but I could not have imagined how profoundly it would shape my worldview and define my karmic path.

It was just me and my then-boyfriend Paul Gleeson, in a 24-foot rowboat. Crossing the ocean demanded an all-consuming focus on a single goal: row towards land and live. We rowed 24 hours a day rotating our shifts every two hours: sleep, row, sleep, row, sleep, row. The only thing sustaining us was freeze-dried food and a desalinator we used to purify our water and hydrate our meals.

For 86 days we rowed through everything: a hurricane, 60-foot swells, sickness, broken bones, and bad sunburns. We had some near-death experiences and yet managed to maintain an optimistic mindset, that is, until one defining event: the breakdown of our desalinator. Without it, we had no food or drinking water.

The dehydration that followed was excruciating—maybe the worst of all the misfortunes we had encountered. I could feel the vitality seeping from every cell in my body. With it went my hope and optimism—the irony of being surrounded by water and not having any water to drink nearly broke me.

When we managed to miraculously repair the desalinator a few days later, I truly appreciated water for the first time in my life. With each cup I drank, I felt spirit flow back into my body. It was a crystallizing moment; I understood how fragile life is, and that water is the foundation of it all.

Back on land, I paid the cost of my adventure at sea. Burnt out and exhausted I could feel that something was off; an internal voice was calling for help. I discovered early cancer cells in my left breast. Despite my great appreciation for Western medicine and gratitude for critical intervention, I knew that it alone wouldn't fully restore my health. My healing journey needed to take a different course.

I decided that my mission to heal was also an opportunity for learning and personal growth so I set out to study holistic nutrition. I sought guidance and mentorship from healers, shamans, herbalists, and naturopaths in books and workshops, and I immersed myself in nature and meditation. When I started connecting the dots between all of the disciplines I was studying, it became clear that hydration was at the base of all wellness practices, just as I had experienced first-hand on that boat.

I started making hydration my priority and combining it with my newfound knowledge of alternative medicine. I started by adding plants, herbs, and adaptogens to my water, which turned my habit of keeping hydrated into an everyday ritual of self-care. A few months into it, I started to notice incremental and profound improvements to my health and wellbeing.

This path I chose worked for me—I eventually found my way back to health, and along the way, realized the power of prioritizing self-care before sick care. Now, my life is about sharing my experience and educating my community about the importance of water and plant-based medicine. I founded Nectar Juicery, an organic cold-pressed juice company in Vancouver, as my first pursuit in nourishing my community.

Here, I am sharing with you the benefits of water and plants that I've been a witness to in my own life. I offer you this book of elixirs as a guide to simple rituals for self-care. It's an invitation to explore your body and discover that wellness can be as simple as connecting to water.

May this book inspire you to move towards greater health, one sip at a time.

—Tori

moving from sick care to self-care

Too often when we think of health we think of something going wrong in the body. But this way of thinking separates our health from our bodies. Your body is not a collection of parts that can go wrong, like a car. Your body has an unbreakable thread of vitality that runs through every part of your being—that thread is your health. When we think of our bodies as whole, we begin to address our health in a new, holistic way.

Your most valuable relationship is the one with your health, because it determines how you show up every day. It will witness every time you fall and pick yourself back up again. It will share your greatest joy and your deepest sorrow. Treat your health with love, like you would a friend, a child, or a partner. Be good to it, as your relationship with the health of your earthly body will only be broken after you breathe your last breath.

As a young person I was taught that medicine should act fast, and that I should expect to feel better immediately. This belief—common to many of us—led me down a path of doing my body more harm than good and diminishing my ability to understand what my body was telling me. Today, I believe all my symptoms of dis-ease are my body giving voice to the attention it is seeking.

When I started taking small, consistent steps toward better health every day, I created a lasting shift in my wellness. I started to hear the signals in my body, alerting me to what my body needed more of or less of. My commitment to incremental improvements to my health deepened my relationship with my body—a relationship I now look forward to investing in daily and preventing sick care by practicing self-care.

When we create momentum by continuing to take steps forward, we inspire more movement and more dynamic energy in our lives. In the context of our health, losing momentum and entering a state of stagnation and inertia can create dis-ease. Take one small step forward every single day and watch your relationship with your health turn to one of wellness.

Water keeps us alive and is essentially the one ritual that we require daily. An elixir is the water you know but made better with plant medicine. Sometimes called tonics or functional waters, elixirs support us on every level—mind, body, and spirit. By adding plants from the earth in the form of herbs, fruits, adaptogens, and superfoods, you are creating water that can support your wellness in incremental, profound ways. The process of creating an elixir is varied—it can be steeped, brewed, or soaked—but the goal of all elixirs is the same: Give your body a consistent source of wellness, and help that wellness flow through you, every day.

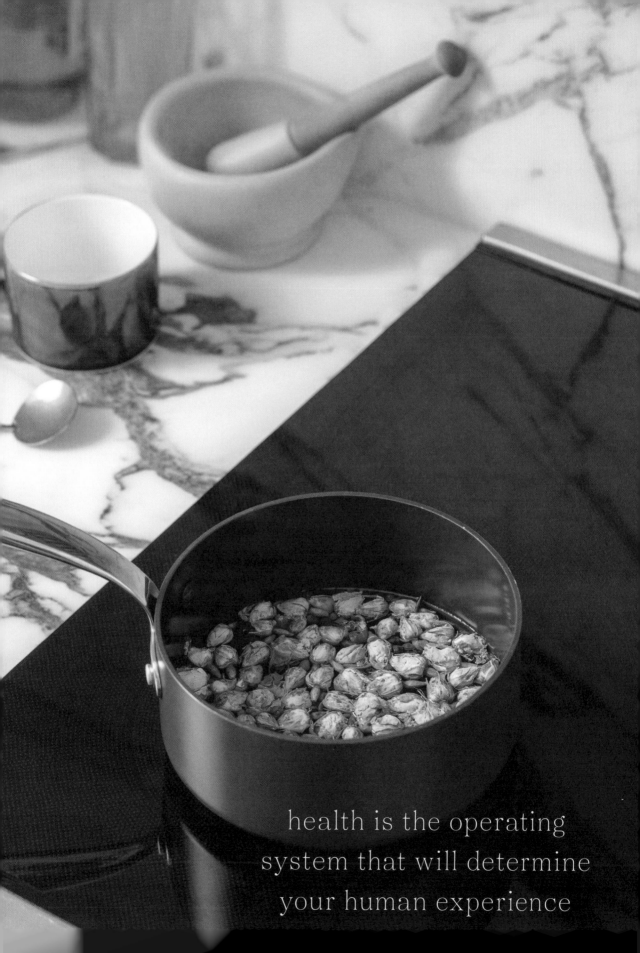

health is the operating
system that will determine
your human experience

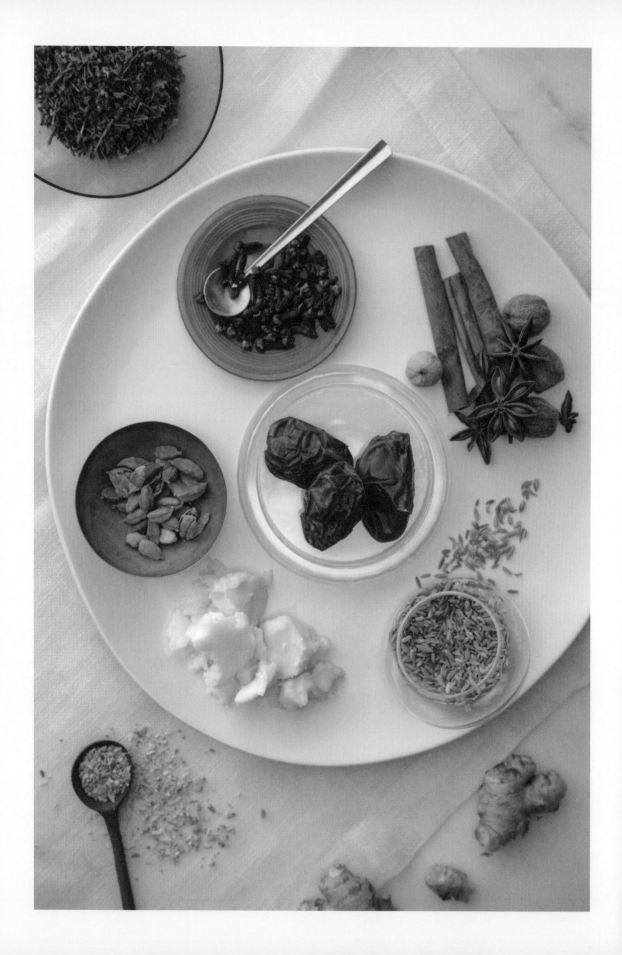

the power of commitment

In order to reap the full wellness benefits of the recipes in this book, I recommend you commit to a few of them at a time. You don't need to go out with an extensive shopping list and buy all the ingredients at once, but instead build your collection of herbs, adaptogens, supplements, and crystals over a lifetime. It's more important to thoughtfully choose the ingredients that support your wellness goals and intentions and get to know their power one recipe at a time.

When you commit to a new ritual, it's helpful to write it down. Whether you track your thoughts in a special notebook or keep notes on your phone, the important thing is to maintain an awareness of the commitment you have made to your health. Ask yourself the following questions each month.

||| overall
How has your wellness been in the last month? Rate it on a scale of 1 to 10, with 10 being you at your most vital and energized. How can you improve your wellness by at least one point?

||| body
How would you describe the current state of your body? Strong, energized, calm, fatigued, uncomfortable, in pain, stressed? How would you like to describe the state of your body?

||| mind
How would you describe the current state of your mental health? Content, apathetic, joyful, melancholic, defeated, inconsistent? What words define your ideal mental state?

||| spirit
How would you describe the current state of your spirit? Aligned, grounded, intuitive, adrift, lost, untethered? What is your spirit calling for?

building a path to wellness

1. set a clear wellness goal
The mind functions best with clarity, and the body functions best when the mind is clear. Reflect on where you want your wellness to be—this is the starting place for developing your wellness goal. Your goal could be anything from energizing your body on a daily basis, to grounding your spirit, or focusing on beauty and rejuvenation from within. Write your goal down.

Get clear on why this wellness goal is important to you and read it daily. This will keep you motivated to maintain your commitment and create new, lifelong rituals.

2. choose your elixirs
There are no wrong choices, since all of the recipes will provide some sort of health benefit, plus you'll be drinking more liquid and staying hydrated through the day. You will see the greatest benefits by committing to one to three recipes that address your wellness goal.

Your wellness goal could be supported by recipes from different chapters. For example, you might want to work on your low energy levels by improving sleep with a recipe from the Sleep chapter (page 43), supercharging your daily routine with a recipe from the Energy chapter (page 91), and boosting your cognitive clarity with a recipe from the Brainpower chapter (page 81).

3. commit to your elixirs for a month at a time
When you commit to change, you commit to improving your life. Drink the elixirs as suggested in the recipe and pay attention to incremental improvements in your wellness.

Stay the course for a full month. I generally drink my elixirs three to five times a week and think of it like taking my internal body to the gym. Use the arrival of each new month as a reminder to check in with your commitment, stay on track, and adjust your elixir choices.

4. reflect on the state of your wellness

Your biggest win will be how consistently you showed up for yourself. Hydrating your body will likely result in improvements to all areas of your wellness. Regardless of your goal, I suspect that you'll be experiencing increased vitality, dewier skin, and smoother digestion after your first 30-day commitment. Reflect on the goal you set for yourself at the beginning of the month and rate your wellness on a 1-to-10 scale again. How would you rank your wellness now? How would you describe the wellness of your body, mind, and spirit?

5. begin the cycle again

The goal of this book is to support you in creating your wellness library over a lifetime. Good health is about momentum, so the more you invest, the better you feel and the easier it gets.

You will feel compelled to use some herbs more so than others, so trust your gut. It is completely fine to put an herb away for a while and come back to it later, just as we do with the spices in our cupboard. One of the main benefits of working with a given herb for a full month is developing an understanding of its taste, texture, and impact on your own individual wellness. This will develop your confidence so that over time, you can start to experiment with them as you do with all your foods and spices. Add them to your favorite curry, soup, coffee; be curious and design your own elixirs to suit your own palate and wellness needs.

questions that may come up

||| should I keep drinking the same elixirs?

If you really love an elixir, and your body says yes, then continue using it! I often like to keep one and change one in my rituals to keep my body moving forward.

||| what if I don't feel better?

That's your body saying no. Not every elixir is for everyone but you will certainly find one that you respond to. Stay curious, keep your intention in mind, and stay attuned to your body's needs and responses.

||| should I change my rituals seasonally?

Many things change seasonally, including our body's natural energy, rhythms, and needs. Most of these recipes can be used year-round, but a few require seasonal ingredients or are best used when needed. Check the recipe descriptions for notes on season-specific uses.

||| what if I take a break?

Plant medicine is best used in small doses over a lifetime. It's okay to come back to it at a different time.

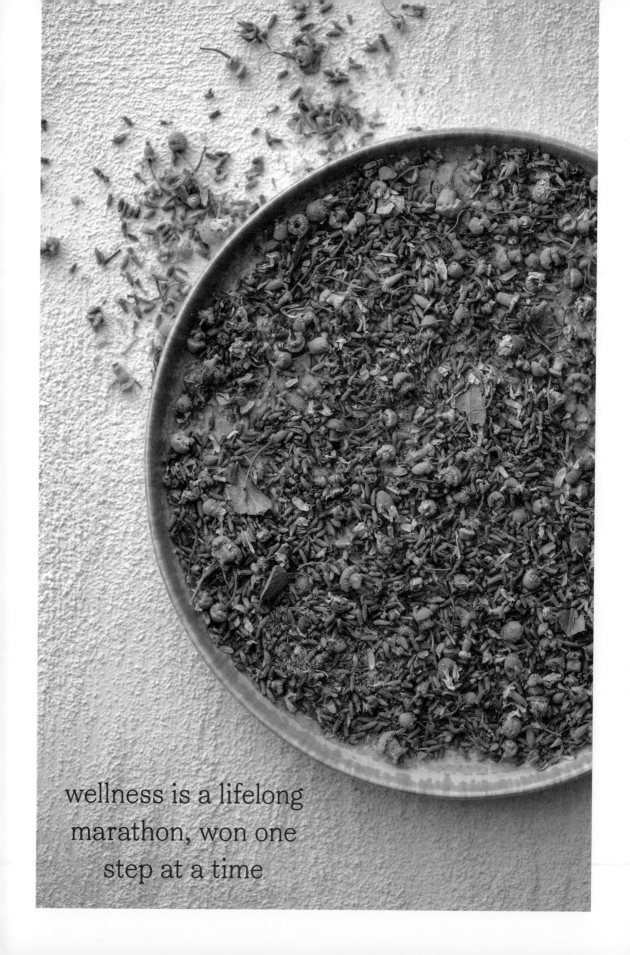

wellness is a lifelong
marathon, won one
step at a time

tips to get you started

accessibility and using what you have

The beauty of creating the elixirs in this book is that you can start with whatever ingredients you can find. Each section includes recipes with simple ingredients you can buy at any grocery store, as well as recipes with ingredients that may take more effort to source but are well worth the investment. For fresh produce, try a grocery store or a farmers' market. For more specialized items, try Amazon or your local health-food store.

To quickly assess recipes you want to start with, I've rated each recipe on a difficulty scale, taking into account how involved the procedure is and whether the ingredients are hard to source. An easy recipe involves only mixing or blending, and uses simple ingredients you can find at a grocery store. A moderate recipe might call for a few more ingredients, involve special tools like a matcha whisk or a French press, or take longer to prepare. An involved recipe might require planning ahead for ingredient sourcing, allowing the drink to rest overnight or longer, or preparing a base for the drink separately—but it's worth it!

||| easy ||| moderate ||| involved

keep it manageable

By choosing two or three recipes at a time to support your specific intention, you are going to optimize your investment in new ingredients, build a relationship with them, and create familiarity around the ritual of making elixirs for your wellness. Different plants require different techniques to maximize their wellness properties. As you build your library of ingredients over time, you will become accustomed to the benefits they offer your body and preparing them. You will eventually think of them as the new salt and pepper.

choose high-quality ingredients

As you build your library of herbs and adaptogens, I highly recommend sourcing the highest-quality ingredients you can find. Whenever possible, buy organic and local to maximize the benefit to your health. Fresh fruits, herbs, and roots should be used seasonally.

Smell and taste herbs and spices before you use them. If they have little or no aroma, they have likely lost their potency and won't support your health.

ingredient substitutions

If you're missing one ingredient, there might be a simple substitution you can use. The elixir may not taste exactly the same, or have identical medicinal properties, but it will be similar enough for you to establish a ritual and start to notice the benefits.

Play with the recipes and tweak them to your palate, as all recipes will have a slightly different outcome, depending on the quality, freshness, and availability of the different ingredients. For a list of ingredients used in this book and available substitutions, see page 132.

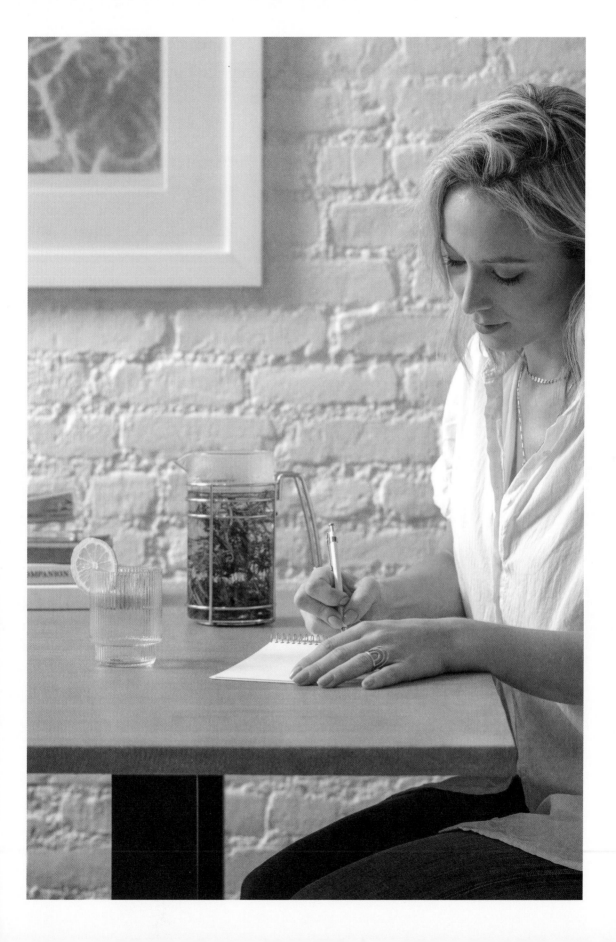

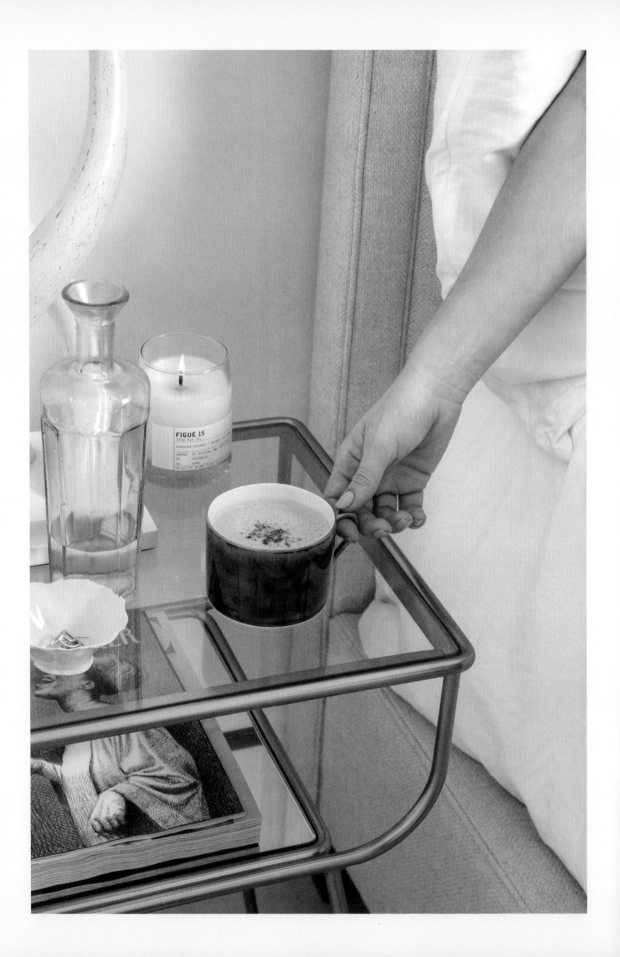

consider the quality of your water

Because water is such a fundamental building block of wellness, how we treat our water is how we treat ourselves. Starting each recipe with pure, fresh water enhances the wellness benefit your body will receive and declares the intention that you are about to create a commitment to your health. For all the recipes in this book, make sure you are using water that is purified and mineralized, and if available, pH balanced.

For a simple way to improve your water quality, purify it with activated charcoal, which will remove chlorine, heavy metals, and other suspended particles, all the while imparting the elemental wellness your body craves. This cost-effective and portable filtration product can be found online—I never travel without one.

use safely

When it comes to plant medicine, more doesn't mean better. Herbs and alternative ingredients are best used consistently in small doses. The elixirs in this book are not meant to treat or cure any form of illness, or replace your current medical treatments, health regimens, or prescriptions. If you are currently taking any other forms of medications, are pregnant, breastfeeding, or have been diagnosed with an illness, I recommend you be your own best advocate, do some research, and consult with your health-care team before adding elixirs to your daily rituals.

essential tools you'll need for most recipes

||| blender (Blendtec or Vitamix)
The incredible power of these blenders will allow you to achieve the creamy textures and emulsifications that the recipes call for.

||| French press
The filtered lid is the ideal tool for removing plant material from your elixir.

||| kettle
Choose a method of boiling water that suits your needs, whether stovetop or electric.

||| measuring utensils and cups
It's important to use the correct amount of the powerful ingredients in elixirs. Make sure you can measure accurately and consistently.

||| quart-size jars with airtight lids
When storing elixirs, it's important to use glass, not plastic, to avoid any unwanted chemicals ending up in the water. Keep the airtight lid sealed when storing to keep aromas of other foods in the refrigerator from affecting your elixir.

||| sacred cup or mug
Choose a cup that feels good in your hands and enhances the quality of your ritual. When you honor the process with a beautiful drinking cup, your mind will shift into a place of greater presence.

||| saucepans with lids, in various sizes
Depending on the volume of the elixir that you will be making, you will need a saucepan large enough to contain the liquid, and a tight-fitting lid.

||| strainer
Many of your elixirs will need to be strained to remove the plant material before you enjoy them. Choose one with a fine-mesh screen to catch all the particles and create the most beautiful elixir.

nice-to-have tools

||| citrus reamer
A reamer is a great way to get every last drop of juice from your citrus fruits, but any method of juicing by hand will work too.

||| frother or hand blender
Some recipes call for a frothy texture but will be just as beneficial without it. In a pinch, use a full-size blender.

||| matcha whisk
This bamboo whisk creates a delicate foam and heightens the ritualistic element of making an elixir. A standard, stainless steel whisk can be used in its place.

||| mortar and pestle
Grinding herbs and spices by hand releases the most potent flavor and medicinal benefits. But you can also use a dedicated spice grinder or coffee grinder.

||| muddler
Bruising leaves to release their delicate oils is a job best done with a muddler. In its place, use a wooden spoon.

||| tea ball infuser
For easy removal of woody and dried plant material, place the solid ingredients inside a tea ball infuser. You can also tie the herbs in a cheesecloth, or strain using a fine-mesh strainer.

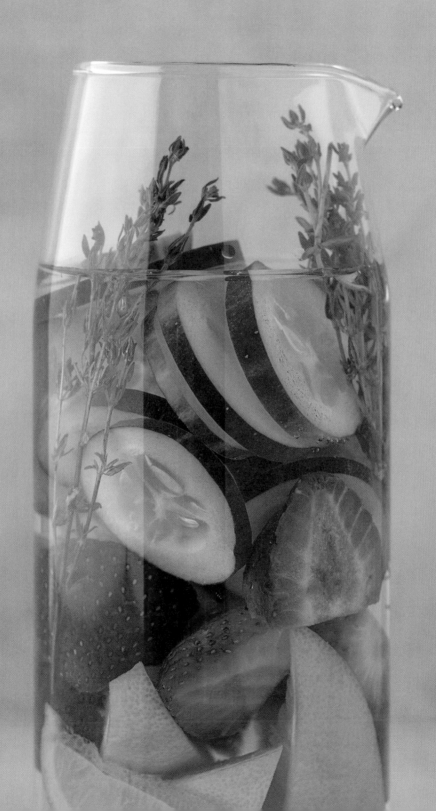

chapter one

listen to your gut and your
body will tell you everything
you need to know

digestion

the gut is the second brain

The place to start, no matter what your wellness goals might be, is investing in your digestion, the foundation of health. Our gut, once thought to be a relatively simple set of organs, is now called our "second brain" because it has so much influence over our body's state. Everything from our skin, immunity, and circulation, to our emotions, strength, and vitality, is improved when our gut health is improved.

I created the following elixirs to give you an efficient way to receive the support your body needs on a daily basis. Two key facets to a healthy gut are allowing rest to promote recovery, and taking in nutrients that can be easily absorbed. Elixirs offer maximum nutrients and require minimal effort by the body for absorption.

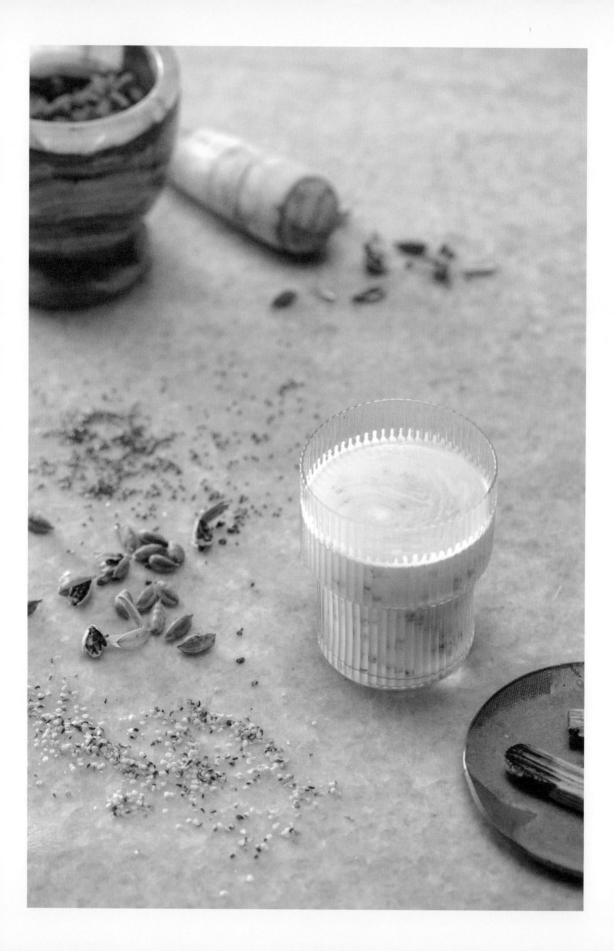

chia
mover

supports the bowels and enhances probiotics

This is a favorite recipe at my juice bar, originally designed as part of a cleansing program to support bowel health and encourage the growth of probiotics in your gut. Try this protein- and fiber-rich elixir and discover the incredible benefit to regulated, healthy bowels. Drinking this handmade hemp milk enhanced with the superfood chia will relieve bloating, discomfort, and irregularity.

Reach for a cup in the early to late afternoon when you're looking for a snack. Support your body even further by drinking in tandem with plenty of water to let the chia work its gut health magic.

makes 4 cups ||| takes 10 minutes ||| rests 2 hours ||| lasts 3 days in the refrigerator

ingredients

||| ½ cup hemp hearts
||| ¼ teaspoon ground cardamom
||| 1 teaspoon ground Ceylon cinnamon or 1 ounce Cinnamon Flow (page 89)
||| ½ teaspoon vanilla extract
||| 4 cups water
||| 2 tablespoons raw honey
||| 1 tablespoon chia seeds

special tools

||| blender
||| quart-size jar with airtight lid

1. In a small bowl, combine the hemp hearts, cardamom, cinnamon, vanilla, and water. Let soak for 1 hour or overnight in the refrigerator.
2. Transfer the mixture to a blender and blend for 3 minutes, or until the liquid looks smooth and you no longer see the black specks from the hemp.
3. Using a fine strainer or a cheesecloth, strain out the solid ingredients pressing down with a spoon to extract all the liquid, then pour the liquid into a quart-size jar. If properly strained, there should be no hemp heart residue or clumps in the jar and the consistency should be smooth and creamy.
4. Add the honey and chia to the jar and stir for 30 seconds.
5. Let sit for 1 hour in the refrigerator. As the chia swells and becomes gelatinous, it may clump. Use a fork to break up the chia before serving.

chia tiny seeds with big benefits

This little superfood is native to Central America and comes from the same plant family as mint. The incredibly high soluble fiber content is what creates the gelatinous substance you see when chia is soaked. This soluble fiber acts like a prebiotic to support the growth of probiotics, and helps you feel fuller by absorbing fluid and expanding in your digestive tract. Add chia to your rituals to support healthy regulation of hunger and bowel movements.

apple cider pre-meal elixir

improves digestive environment

This was the first remedy I learned while studying holistic nutrition. What stuck with me was the discovery of wisdom in our everyday foods that we can access when we know how to work with them. This simple apple cider elixir naturally neutralizes stomach acid, acting as a probiotic and helping our bodies digest food efficiently.

Drink it 15 to 20 minutes before each meal to help prevent constipation and relieve bloating. You can also supercharge this recipe and make it an herbal vinegar. Fill a quarter of a quart-size jar with your favorite dry herbs (I love using nettle for this), top with warm apple cider vinegar, and seal. Let sit for up to 2 weeks, then add a tablespoon daily to your salad, water, or favorite beverage.

makes 1 cup ||| takes 2 minutes ||| best consumed immediately

ingredients

||| 1 to 2 tablespoons unpasteurized apple cider
vinegar with mother
||| 2 cups water

1. Mix the vinegar with 1 cup water.
2. Use the remaining water to swish around your mouth between sips, to prevent the vinegar affecting your tooth enamel and irritating your esophagus.

apple cider vinegar the mother of all vinegars

Created from crushed, fermented apples, apple cider vinegar (ACV) is very high in acetic acid, which is known to kill pathogens like bacteria. Some studies show that taking ACV can help balance blood sugar levels, reduce cholesterol levels, and support a healthy blood pressure. The murky appearance and the "mother" found in organic, unfiltered ACV are caused by strands of naturally-occurring masses of proteins, enzymes, and beneficial bacteria.

ginger soother

soothes digestion

I discovered the benefits of ginger while crossing the Atlantic Ocean, when I turned to fresh ginger as a way to naturally soothe seasickness. This ancient root is an all-around digestive superstar, as it relieves nausea, bloating, and constipation, and also prepares the body for receiving and absorbing nutrients. The addition of German chamomile creates the perfect balance between supporting and soothing actions.

Sip 1 cup twice a day to relieve digestive upset, and 20 minutes before eating to prepare the body for digestion. Ginger is stimulating, so those who easily overheat should use it in moderation.

Health tip: Do not use this recipe if suffering from colitis, ulcers, or an overactive stomach.

makes 4 cups ||| takes 30 minutes ||| lasts 4 days in the refrigerator

ingredients

||| 1 (4- to 5-inch) piece fresh ginger root, grated
||| 4 cups water
||| 4 tablespoons dried German chamomile
||| juice of 1 to 2 lemons
||| raw honey or stevia to taste

special tools

||| grater
||| quart-size jar with airtight lid

1. In a medium saucepan, combine the ginger and water, then cover and bring to a boil. Reduce heat to low and simmer for 10 minutes.
2. Remove from heat, add the chamomile, and let steep for 15 minutes.
3. Using a strainer, strain out the solid ingredients, then pour the liquid into a quart-size jar.
4. Add the lemon juice and honey.
5. Serve immediately or store in the refrigerator in an airtight jar. Before drinking, warm slightly or allow to return to room temperature. This elixir should not be consumed cold.

German chamomile   the mother healer

German chamomile, more commonly available than Roman chamomile, has been used to soothe digestive problems for thousands of years. This tiny flower contains a chemical compound called spiroether, which is a strong antispasmodic and eases tense muscles and intestines. Using this herb regularly can help with troubles like indigestion, acidity, gastritis, bloating, colic, Crohn's disease, and irritable bowel syndrome. It is so gentle that it is suitable for children.

cumin coriander fennel reset

supports digestion between meals

This personal favorite is sometimes known simply as CCF, a combination that is also an Ayurvedic staple. There is a strong link between the brain and the gut—the key to healing the body is to support the digestive system. This broth-like elixir gently kindles the digestive fire *agni* and burns the source of dis-ease *amma*, all without aggravating any body types.

Keep this elixir on hand in your home at all times and drink 1 cup between meals to avoid snacking, stimulate the digestive tract, help break down natural toxins, and encourage assimilation of nutrients. I make this recipe once a week and take one shot a day to keep my digestion optimal.

Health tip: Be careful with this elixir if you have diabetes, as cumin and coriander can lower blood sugar.

makes 4 cups ||| takes 20 minutes ||| lasts 3 days in the refrigerator

ingredients

||| 1 tablespoon cumin seeds
||| 1 tablespoon fennel seeds
||| 1 tablespoon coriander seeds
||| 4 cups water
||| 1 tablespoon dried German chamomile (optional)
||| 1 teaspoon maple syrup (optional)

special tools

||| quart-size jar with airtight lid

1. In a medium saucepan, combine the cumin, fennel, and coriander seeds, and toast until fragrant.
2. Add the water and bring to a rolling boil for 5 minutes.
3. Remove from heat and add in the chamomile (if using). Let steep for 10 minutes.
4. Using a strainer, strain out the solid ingredients, then pour the liquid into a quart-size jar.
5. Add the maple syrup (if using) and stir.
6. Serve hot or cold.

CCF power in numbers

Also known as Ayurveda's miracle tea, CCF is a combination of three seeds with powerful abilities to soothe digestive troubles. Cumin seeds can help reduce cramps, gas, and indigestion. Coriander seeds soothe an overly acidic stomach and skin rashes, and relieve joint pain. Fennel seeds stimulate appetite and relieve cramping and gas.

triphala trifecta

resets digestion overnight

My introduction to Ayurvedic medicine was when I first took triphala while in Bangladesh, to deal with an out-of-sorts digestive system. I've kept this elixir straightforward, as I learned it from my *ayah* (house mother). Make an overnight investment in your digestion—the key player in the body—by accessing the incredible benefits of triphala. This antioxidant-rich elixir helps to strengthen the digestive system, so your body is better able to complete the detoxification cycle, absorb nutrients, and recover.

Sip 30 to 60 minutes before bed and take your gut to the gym while you sleep. Triphala's unique tannin taste is indicative of its intense benefits, so 1 cup is as much as should be enjoyed in a day.

makes 1 cup ||| takes 10 minutes ||| lasts 5 days in the refrigerator

ingredients

||| 1 cup water
||| ¼ teaspoon triphala powder
||| 1 German chamomile or lavender tea bag (optional for flavor)

special tools

||| matcha whisk

1. Bring the water to a boil.
2. Scoop the triphala into a cup and pour a small amount of hot water over it, then use a matcha whisk to emulsify until smooth.
3. Add the tea bag (if using) and the remaining water and let steep for 5 minutes.

note: Triphala's strong tannin taste is key to supporting digestion. For best results, avoid sweeteners of any kind.

triphala   three times the synergy

A combination of three dried fruits (*amalaki, bibhitaki,* and *haritaki*), triphala powder has been used for thousands of years in Ayurvedic medicine to move the body to receiving mode. It is considered tridoshic and therefore supportive of every body type. The synergy of the three fruits has a gentle yet deeply rejuvenating and balancing influence on the digestive system and represents five out of the six Ayurvedic tastes. Triphala is especially rich in gallic acid, ellagic acid, and chebulinic acid, all of which are antioxidants that support the entire body.

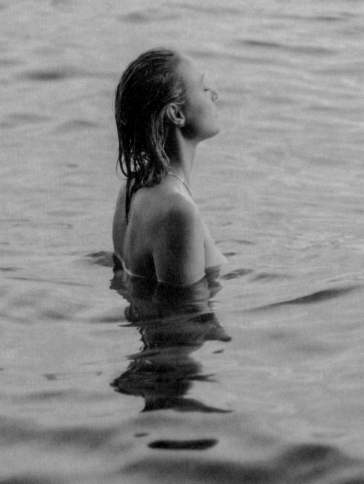

chapter two

the state of our external
body reflects the state of
our internal body

beauty

an inside job

When we think of physical beauty, we often focus on external attributes, like dewy skin, lustrous hair, and bright eyes. Of course, hydration plays a key role in all of them, which means beauty starts on the inside. Achieving true beauty requires taking in enough nutrients and water to support your largest organ: the skin. When you're well hydrated and your mineral levels are optimal, your cells are thoroughly oxygenated, and you exude more pheromones. You literally have the *it* factor.

Bring your inner and outer beauty into alignment by accessing medicinal plant wisdom, the way our ancestors did for thousands of years. Use these elixirs to protect your skin from free radicals and loss of elasticity.

collagen tight

hydrates and tightens

I've been serving this at my juicery for years—it's a favorite for increasing skin elasticity and vibrancy. The vitamin C in hibiscus paired with the vital protein collagen creates the foundation for healthy, glowing skin.

When it comes to this drink, consistency is key—drink 1 cup daily before lunch for a minimum of 6 weeks to notice results.

makes 4 cups ||| takes 30 minutes ||| rests 1 hour ||| lasts 5 days in the refrigerator

ingredients

||| 4 cups water
||| 2 tablespoons dried hibiscus flowers
||| 1 tablespoon dried Schisandra berries
||| 2 tablespoons marine collagen
||| 1½ tablespoons raw honey, or to taste
||| Himalayan salt to taste
||| Bulgarian rose water (optional)

special tools

||| French press
||| quart-size jar with airtight lid

1. Bring the water to a boil.
2. In a French press, combine the hibiscus and Schisandra berries, and cover with boiling water. Let steep for 20 minutes, then press down the filter.
3. Place the collagen in a quart-size jar and add 2 to 3 tablespoons of the liquid from the French press.
4. Using a fork, mix the collagen until smooth and emulsified, adding more liquid as needed.
5. Pour the remaining liquid from the French press into the jar.
6. Add the honey and salt, then seal the jar with a lid.
7. Allow to cool for at least 1 hour in the refrigerator. Before drinking, shake gently to recombine the collagen, which may naturally separate and settle.
8. For a special treat, add 2 tablespoons of rose water per cup.

collagen a time-honored Japanese beauty secret

Collagen is the foundation of smooth, youthful-looking skin; it's the most important structural protein in the body. It represents 75 percent of our skin, and as we move past our twenties, we start losing about 1 percent of our collagen per year. Diminishing levels of collagen give way to inflammation in the body, resulting in the typical signs of aging. Consuming collagen daily will strengthen hair and nails, as well as prevent joint pain and the formation of fine lines. Look for marine collagen (also known as fish collagen) for the most bioavailable source of collagen for your body.

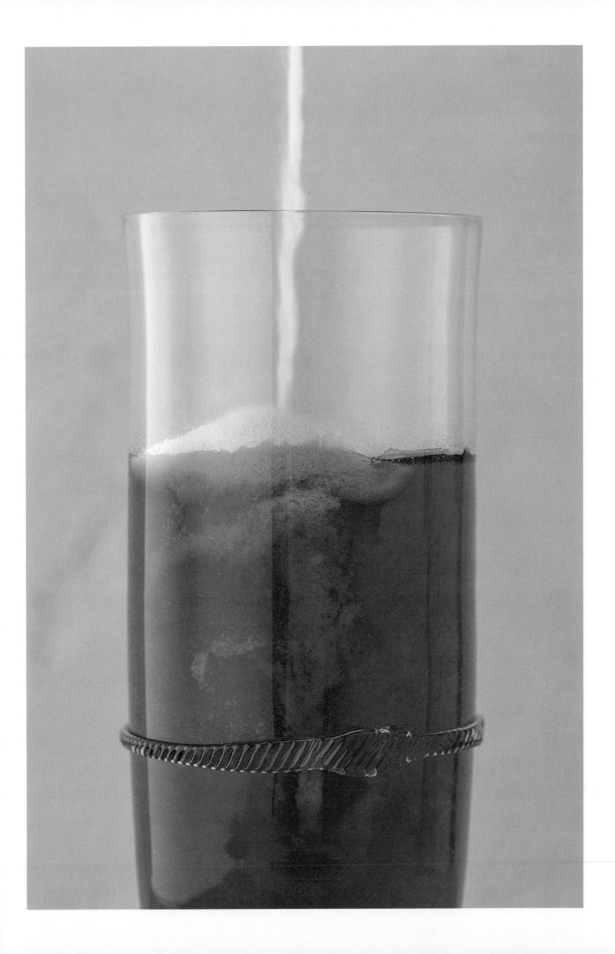

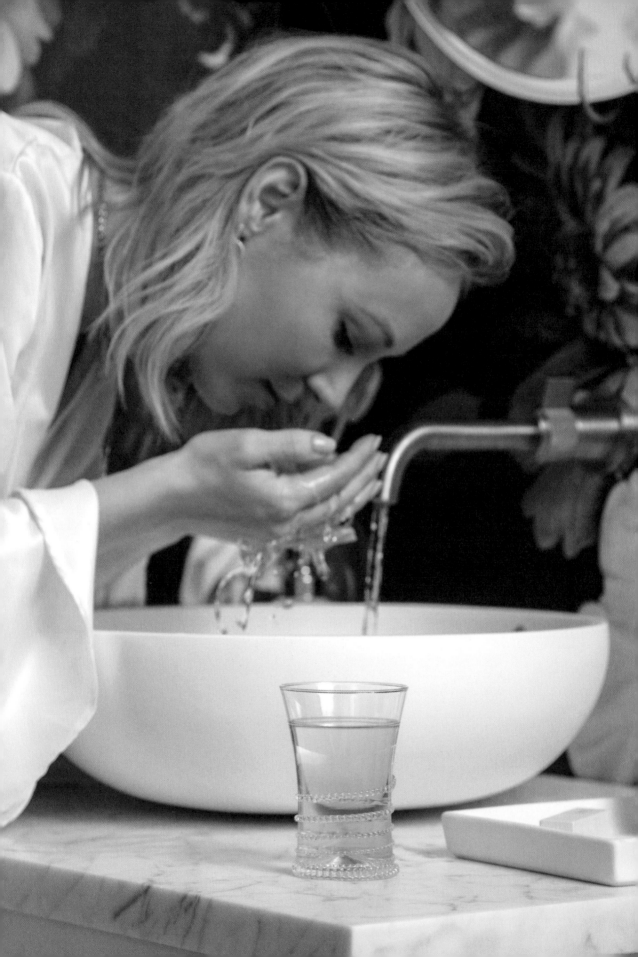

rose bright

brightens skin

This elixir made with skin-brightening rose was my first-ever daily ritual and investment in self-care. All plants have a vibration frequency, and rose vibrates at the highest frequency of all plant essences. When you add it to your water, you take in the benefits of its vibration. Schisandra berry is one of my favorite adaptogens and helps my mind feel expansive and bright. While sipping this as I prepare for my day, I feel supported and aligned—like I'm giving my body a hug. When I start my mornings this way, I am able to stand in a place of self-love and give myself permission to shine from the inside out.

Health tip: If using pharmaceutical drugs or treating illness, consult with your doctor before consuming Schisandra berry. It is not recommended for those with a cold or the flu, or for those with pre-existing illnesses.

makes 1½ cups ||| takes 40 minutes ||| lasts 7 days in the refrigerator

ingredients

- ||| 1 cup fresh rose petals or ½ cup dried (food grade)
- ||| 1 tablespoon dried Schisandra berries
- ||| 2 cups water
- ||| Himalayan salt
- ||| 1 tablespoon Bulgarian rose water (optional)

special tools

- ||| quart-size jar with airtight lid

1. In a medium saucepan, combine the rose petals and Schisandra berries.
2. Add the water to the saucepan and bring to a boil.
3. Reduce to low heat and simmer for 30 minutes, or until the petals have faded.
4. Using a strainer, strain out the solid ingredients, then pour the liquid into a quart-size jar. Add a pinch of salt, and the rose water (if using).
5. Seal with a lid and store in the refrigerator.
6. To serve, add 3 tablespoons of the elixir to 1 cup water and sip.

note: The flavor of this elixir is bright and astringent, so avoid sweeteners of any kind.

rose the beauty queen

Rose has been a symbol of love, beauty, and internal healing for centuries. For more than 400 years, central Bulgaria has been home to the Rose Valley. Rich with ideal soil, and the perfect level of humidity, the valley produces the world's highest-quality, highest-vibrational roses. These roses are the source of precious rose otto, an essential oil prized for its anti-inflammatory, skin-soothing, and beautifying and brightening qualities. For a higher-vibration drink, add 1 tablespoon of Bulgarian rose water to your concentrate. Make sure you source a pure concentrate made without glycerin.

nettle
glow

regenerates skin

The key to lasting hydration is all about taking in the right amount of minerals. I use this fresh, astringent elixir to help my body reach optimal mineral levels and maintain hydration. Nettle and sea buckthorn create a nutrient-dense elixir that will keep you feeling youthful all day by detoxifying your system and cleansing your palate, without a touch of sting.

Make this recipe in the evening, so you can sip on it the following day. As most of us are deficient in minerals, this is also a helpful recovery elixir after your body goes through extreme stress, like hiking or even giving birth.

makes 4 cups ||| takes 40 minutes ||| rests overnight ||| lasts 5 days in the refrigerator

ingredients

||| 4 cups water
||| 1 cup fresh stinging nettle leaves or
   ½ cup dried
||| 4 tablespoons fresh sea buckthorn
   berries or 3 tablespoons dried
||| ½ cup packed fresh mint leaves
||| 5 slices English cucumber

special tools

||| French press
||| protective gloves (if using fresh nettle)
||| quart-size jar with airtight lid

1. Bring the water to a boil.
2. In a French press, combine the nettle, sea buckthorn, and mint. (Make sure to wear protective gloves when handling fresh nettle.)
3. Cover with the boiling water and let steep for 20 minutes, then press down the filter.
4. Pour the elixir into a quart-size jar and allow to cool.
5. Add in the cucumber, seal with a lid, and store in the refrigerator overnight.

stinging nettle forest defender

Sometimes known simply as nettle, this plant has acid-filled cells on its stems and leaves to protect against being consumed by forest animals. Nettles are packed with minerals our body depends on to function, like calcium, potassium, silicic acid, and iron. Consuming nettle is known to support healthy skin, nails, and hair, and it is a potent diuretic that can relieve puffiness.

tocos royal jelly plumper

protects and moisturizes

I turn to this recipe in the winter when my skin gets dry and I use this youth-enhancing elixir as a drink for internal moisturizing. Find your perfect balance with royal jelly, known for its antibacterial support, and moisturizing tocos, which provides the creamy texture and is a source of highly bioavailable vitamin E, one of the foundations of healthy skin.

Drink this in the evening as often as you desire to nourish your skin inside and out. Once a week, try making a paste of a few tablespoons of tocos and water, then rub into your skin—it's like food for your face.

makes 1 cup ||| takes 20 minutes ||| best consumed immediately

ingredients

||| 1¼ cups water
||| 1 tablespoon dried German chamomile
||| 1 tablespoon Ceylon cinnamon chips
||| 2 tablespoons tocos powder
||| 1½ teaspoons royal jelly or raw honey, or to taste
||| Ground Ceylon cinnamon, for sprinkling
||| ½ cup ice, for serving (optional)

special tools

||| blender

1. In a medium saucepan, bring the water to a boil. Add the chamomile and cinnamon chips, then reduce heat, cover, and simmer for 15 minutes.
2. Using a strainer, strain out the solid ingredients, then pour the liquid into a blender.
3. Add the tocos and royal jelly, then blend on high until frothy.
4. Pour into a mug and sprinkle with cinnamon before serving. For a cold drink, pour over ice.

tocos nature's dairy-free creamer

Tocos, or rice bran solubles, gets its unique name from tocopherols, which is the form of vitamin E found in this supplement. To create tocos, the shell that surrounds a grain of rice is ground to a fine powder so that we can benefit from its highly absorbable vitamin E, which is incredibly important in developing connective tissue and muscle and supports the body's natural detoxification process.

calendula calmer

reduces inflammation

Spending a day at the beach by the beautiful ocean is something I love to do, but it can result in red and irritated skin. This elixir is the perfect after-beach care regimen—the calendula will soothe the redness, while the burdock will address the underlying inflammation. Naturally, I like to serve this drink over ice.

You can drink 1 cup daily during beach season to ease inflammation and support tissue healing, or when skin is showing extra redness. Double the benefits by dabbing on irritated skin with a cotton pad.

the base: makes 4 cups ||| takes 25 minutes ||| rests 24 hours ||| lasts 7 days in the refrigerator
the elixir: makes 1 cup ||| takes 3 minutes ||| best consumed immediately

ingredients

for the base
||| 1 teaspoon dried burdock root
||| 4 cups water
||| 4 tablespoons dried calendula flowers

for the elixir
||| 1 teaspoon MCT oil
||| raw honey or stevia to taste
||| ½ cup ice, for serving (optional)

special tools
||| quart-size jar with airtight lid
||| blender

To make the base
1. In a medium saucepan, combine the burdock and water, and bring to a boil.
2. Reduce to low heat, cover, and simmer for 10 minutes.
3. Place the calendula in a quart-size jar, then add the burdock and water.
4. Steep for 15 minutes, then seal with a lid and let sit in the refrigerator for 24 hours.
5. Using a strainer, strain out the solid ingredients, and pour the liquid back into the jar.
6. Keep in the refrigerator for up to a week and use as the base for your elixir.

To make the elixir
1. In a blender, combine 1 cup of the base with the MCT oil and honey.
2. Blend until frothy, then serve. For a cold drink, pour over ice.

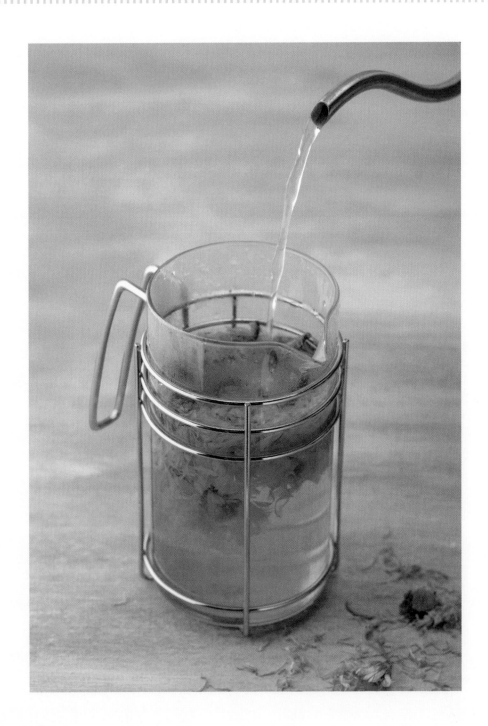

calendula the sunshine healer

Sunny and cheerful calendula is from the same plant family as daisies and marigolds but comes packed with anti-inflammatory and other healing properties. Calendula has been used to soothe the skin and the digestive tract, detoxify the body, prevent infections, and encourage the body to heal itself. Taken orally or used topically, the benefits of calendula have been tried and tested for thousands of years.

chapter three

connect the cycles of
your body with the
cycles of the earth

sleep

find your rhythm

So much of our ability to thrive is connected to our ability to sleep. Sleep is not a nice-to-have luxury—it's a necessity for living to our full potential. It's a natural part of our daily rhythm and allows our brain and body to not only rest, but also to take in, process, and store all the information our senses collected throughout the day. The rising of the sun and the moon cues our bodies to wake and rest, and the wisdom of plant medicine can help us tap into our own body's rhythms to find deep, consistent, and life-enhancing sleep.

Sometimes our modern lives leave us sleep-deprived and in need of help in achieving our best slumber—the following recipes can help bring rejuvenating rest and a good bedtime ritual back into our lives. Establish a ritual by sipping an elixir while you unwind and prepare for sleep, whether that means tapping into your subconscious, calming your nervous system, or addressing sleeplessness.

ashwagandha
chai calmer

relieves stress before bed

Ashwagandha is my favorite herb of all time—I would recommend this great herb to start with and develop into a staple. I use it to regulate the effects of daily stress on my body. Ashwagandha works by balancing cortisol, a stress hormone which can cause sleep disturbances. Cortisol levels are meant to follow our circadian rhythms and naturally decrease in the early evening in preparation for sleep. When life is taking a toll on my ability to rest and recover, I sip this and ask ashwagandha to step in as my sleep ally.

Create a bedtime ritual by sipping this drink in the evening before turning out the lights.

makes 2 cups ||| takes 30 minutes ||| best consumed immediately

ingredients

- 3 pitted dates
- 1 (1½-inch) piece fresh ginger, sliced or grated
- 1 Ceylon cinnamon stick or 1 tablespoon chips
- 2 star anise pods
- 1 teaspoon fennel seeds

- 4 cloves
- ¼ teaspoon grated nutmeg
- 1 tablespoon cardamom pods
- 2 teaspoons ashwagandha bark or powder
- 2 tablespoons dried tulsi (optional)

- 3 cups water
- 2 tablespoons coconut butter
- 1 teaspoon vanilla extract
- Himalayan salt

special tools

- blender

1. Soak the dates in warm water until soft, then drain and set aside.
2. Combine the ginger, cinnamon, star anise, fennel, cloves, nutmeg, cardamom, ashwagandha, tulsi (if using), and water in a saucepan and bring to a boil.
3. Cover and simmer for 20 minutes, then remove from heat.
4. Using a strainer, strain out the solid ingredients then pour the liquid into a blender. Add the soaked dates, coconut butter, vanilla, and a pinch of salt.
5. Blend until the dates are smooth and the beverage is creamy.

ashwagandha the ultimate adaptogen

This Ayurvedic herb is one of the most powerful adaptogens and nervines on the planet. It balances the adrenal system, regulates overall hormone levels, and supports the body and mind through stressful times. Studies are showing that it is an effective remedy for anxiety and stress, while lowering cortisol levels and supporting the brain.

valerian wind-down

calms sleeplessness and excitability

When you're a little too wound up this elixir can help you wind down, calm your nerves, and settle into your deepest slumber. Valerian is a powerful natural sedative, while lavender has been used for centuries to induce general calm. I use this when I'm wired, overtired, and really need to get some rest.

Consistency is key when dealing with insomnia and establishing a bedtime ritual. Sip 1 cup 30 minutes before bedtime daily to relax into sleep mode.

Health tip: Do not use valerian before driving or partaking in any activity that requires alertness.

makes 2 cups ||| takes 10 minutes ||| best consumed immediately

ingredients

||| 2 cups water
||| 1 tablespoon dried lavender
||| 1 tablespoon dried valerian root
||| 1 tablespoon dried German chamomile

special tools

||| French press

1. Bring the water to a boil.
2. In a French press, combine the lavender, valerian root, and chamomile, and cover with the boiling water. Let steep for 5 minutes, then press down the filter.

note: Avoid sweetening this elixir to help your body wind down.

valerian nature's sedative

This root is a potent nervine and is used to promote deep relaxation and to aid with sleep disorders, anxiety, and physiological stress. It contains valerenic acid, a compound which helps with relaxation and calmness of the mind.

tulsi
hot toddy

balances the mind

I created this calming, non-alcoholic, herbal rendition of the traditional hot toddy and added tulsi, an Ayurvedic staple. This soothing, warming elixir supports a balanced mind and calms the gut.

When you feel anxiety coming on and are seeking a sense of ease, sip on this drink to unwind. Drink two to three times a week to feel supported and relaxed.

makes 1 cup ||| takes 20 minutes ||| best consumed immediately

ingredients

||| 1 cup water
||| 1 tablespoon dried tulsi
||| ¼ teaspoon ashwagandha bark (optional)
||| 2 teaspoons fresh lemon juice
||| 2 teaspoons raw honey
||| 1 lemon slice, for garnish
||| 5 whole cloves, for garnish

special tools

||| tea ball infuser
||| teapot

1. Bring the water to a boil.
2. Fill a tea ball infuser with the tulsi and ashwagandha (if using). Place the infuser into a teapot.
3. Pour the boiling water into the teapot and let steep, covered, for 15 minutes.
4. Remove the infuser and mix in the lemon juice and honey.
5. Serve in a cup with a floating lemon slice pierced with the cloves.
6. Sip this drink hot.

tulsi earthly goddess

Also known as holy basil, this adaptogenic variety of basil is an herbal medicine staple, and is an essential part of the worship of the Hindu god, Vishnu. Sometimes called "the herb for all reasons," tulsi is used to support a balanced mind, good digestion, and lowered stress levels. Its antibacterial properties are used in the treatment of respiratory and skin conditions, and for soothing insect bites.

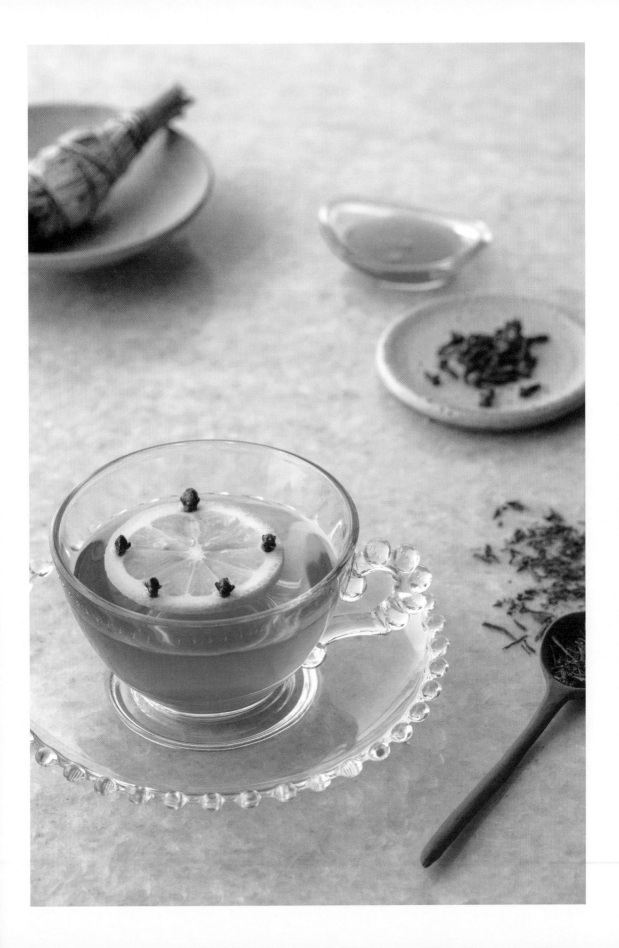

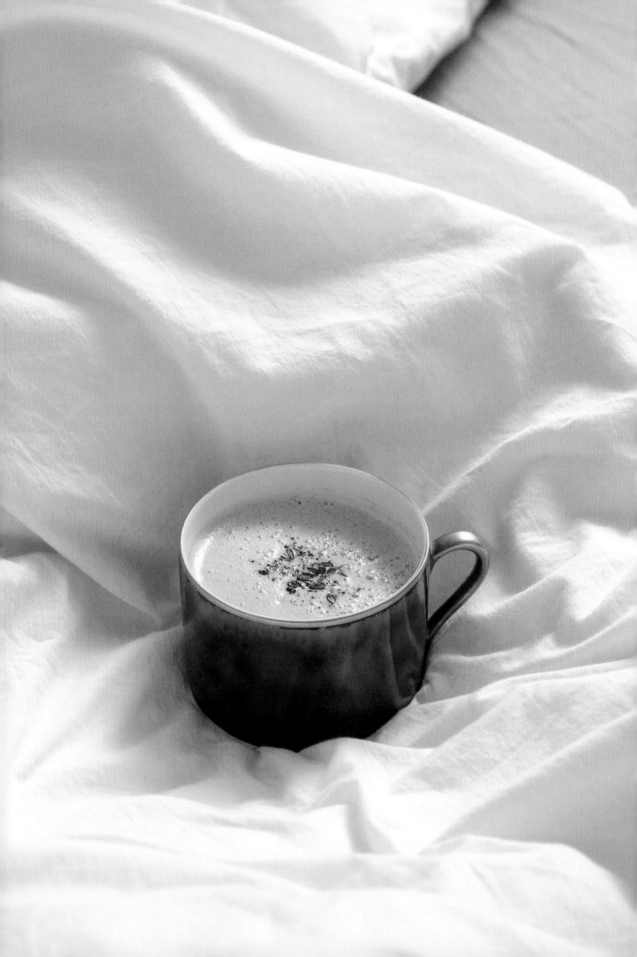

mugwort dreamer

aids lucid dreaming

Mugwort has produced some of the most fascinating and lucid dreaming experiences of my entire life. This is my favorite way to set up for slumber and prepare to process the day. Sometimes what we're not ready to see in our waking state comes to us in our dream state.

Sip 1 cup 30 to 60 minutes before bed and set your dream intention. Make sure your surroundings are quiet, the lights are dimmed, and you're relaxed. On nights that you try this, please take this one piece of advice: Buckle up.

Health tip: As it can also encourage menstruation, avoid this potent herb if you are pregnant, or even attempting to get pregnant.

makes 1 cup ||| takes 5 minutes ||| best consumed immediately

ingredients

||| 1 cup water
||| 1 teaspoon dried mugwort
||| 1 tablespoon coconut butter
||| 2 teaspoons raw honey, or to taste

special tools

||| blender

1. Bring the water to a boil.
2. Pour the boiling water into a blender and add the mugwort, coconut butter, and honey.
3. Blend until the mugwort is smooth.
4. Serve in a sacred cup.

mugwort total dream recall

Sometimes confused with wormwood, mugwort was used by sailors as tobacco when they ran out or wanted a change in their day—or perhaps their night. It is often used for general relaxation and to encourage vivid, lucid dreams and the ability to recall them in the morning.

chapter four

tune in and
build resilience

stress management

take a proactive approach

The effects of stress on the body create inflammation, demineralization, dehydration, fatigue, toxicity, and many other health concerns. The key to managing stress is not allowing it to get to a tipping point where it results in dis-ease. Maintain a healthy conversation with the stress in your body by investing in your inner peace daily. I designed the following recipes to be equal parts joyful and beneficial, and to ultimately keep your body out of survival mode, so you can recover and develop resilience.

Water-based elixirs are a powerful way to speak to the body, because water is the conduit for all cellular life on Earth; plants and animals alike—we can't survive long without it. When you are stressed, your body needs the most hydration support—stress is a dehydrator, and dehydration causes stress, creating the perfect storm. Establish a daily ritual by sipping an elixir and checking in with your body. At the end of a stressful day, reconnecting with wellness can be as simple as elevating the water you drink and sipping your way to a state of balance and calm.

Schisandra berry 5-flavor

increases zest for life

Schisandra berry is one of my absolute favorites and a staple in my home. I turn to it so often it feels like I'm in a long-term relationship with this adaptogen. It has a flavor like no other berry and it has a special place in my rituals for baseline wellness. The five tastes, referred to in Chinese medicine and mostly unfamiliar to our Western palates, are what help tonify and balance our bodies.

I take this elixir to help counteract the effects of daily stresses, reduce inflammation in my body, and open up my perspective to my ability to thrive. Sip 1 cup every day as an all-encompassing investment in your daily wellness.

Health tip: This elixir is not recommended if you are already feeling unwell, taking prescription drugs, or pregnant.

makes 4 cups ||| takes 25 minutes ||| lasts 2 days in the refrigerator

ingredients

||| 4 cups water
||| 1 teaspoon dried Schisandra berries
||| 2 sprigs lemon balm or mint
||| ½ grapefruit, halved
||| 1 teaspoon maple syrup, plus more to taste

special tools

||| muddler
||| quart-size jar with airtight lid

1. In a medium saucepan, combine the water and Schisandra berries, and bring to a boil.
2. Reduce to low heat and simmer for 15 to 20 minutes. (Don't cook longer than 20 minutes as the berries can become bitter the longer you cook them.) Let cool.
3. Using a muddler, muddle the lemon balm in the bottom of a quart-size jar, then squeeze in the grapefruit juice and drop the rinds into the jar.
4. Using a strainer, strain out the solid ingredients, then add the liquid to the jar. Let rest for a few minutes.
5. Stir in the maple syrup and serve.

Schisandra berry *the ultimate berry*

Called Wu Wei Zi, or "the five-flavor berry," Schisandra is a fruit used as a food and as an adaptogenic medicine. Chinese medicine assumes the existence of five tastes in our digestion, each of which is effective at treating different body systems. Schisandra contains all five, making it highly beneficial to the entire body. It is taken to increase resilience to stress, to boost energy, and support physical endurance, which is why it is often served to Chinese athletes before competition.

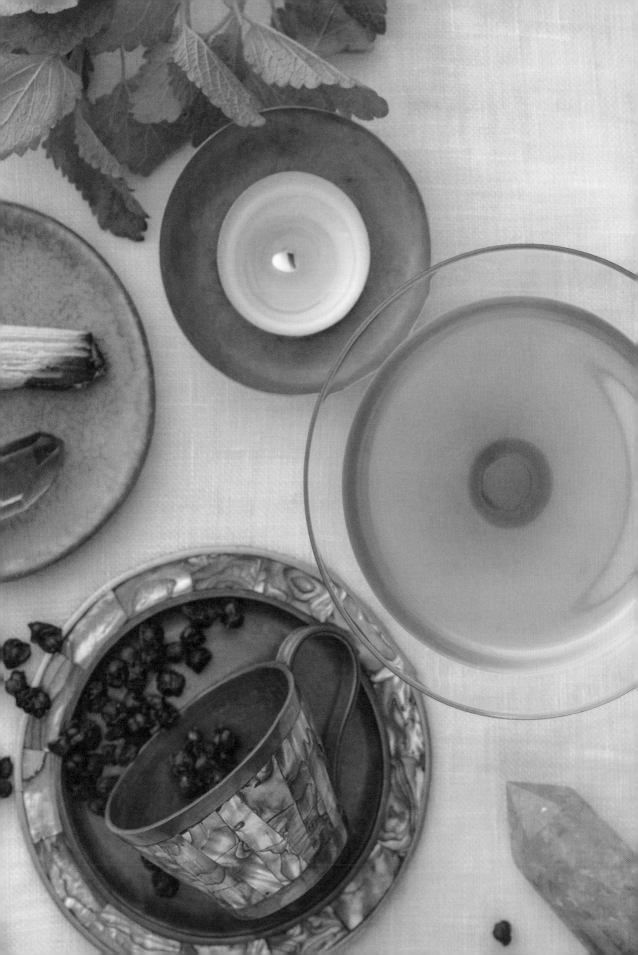

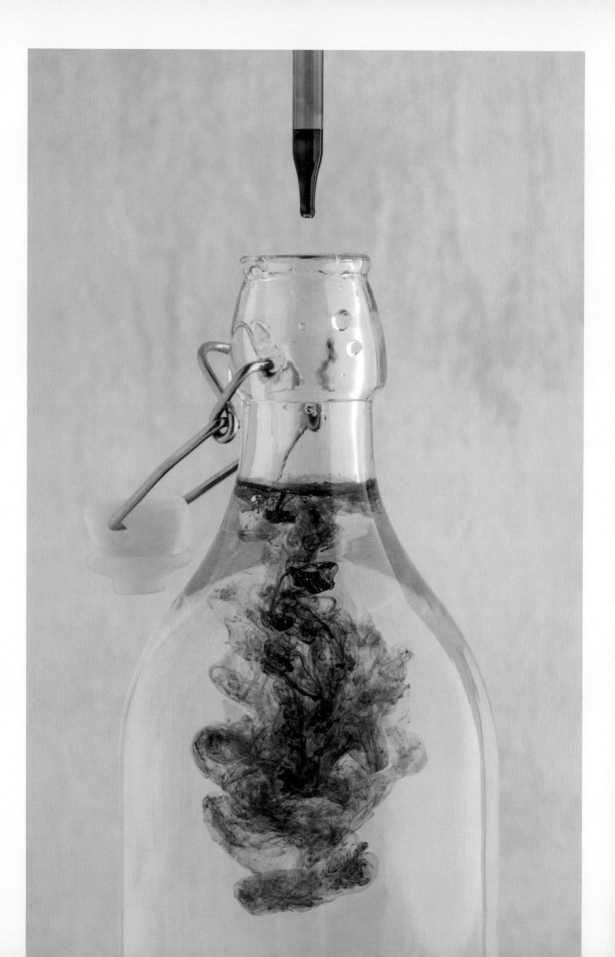

chlorophyll lemonade

aids recovery from physical stress

Chlorophyll is essentially the life-giving matter in plants and it has an amazing ability to build up our blood and vitality, too. Consuming chlorophyll gives us energy and supports the body's ability to heal and recover by increasing the number of red bloods cells, which are key in transporting oxygen to the heart. I like to combine chlorophyll with lemon and maple syrup in this elixir to create a sports drink with an all-natural, vibrant color. Be mindful of countertops, fabrics, and hands when using chlorophyll, as it may stain them.

Pour into your favorite cup, once a day, and visualize your body as a thriving plant, accessing the energy of the sun to grow.

makes 4½ cups ||| takes 2 minutes ||| lasts 4 days in the refrigerator

ingredients

||| 4 cups water
||| 4 teaspoons liquid chlorophyll
||| Himalayan salt
||| juice of 1 lemon
||| maple syrup to taste

special tools

||| quart-size jar with airtight lid

1. In a quart-size jar, combine all the ingredients. Stir, or seal with a lid and shake until combined.
2. If not serving immediately, keep refrigerated in an airtight jar.

chlorophyll the liquid sunshine

Plants use chlorophyll to create food, and humans use chlorophyll to create medicine that can help our bodies recover faster. Green plants harness the energy of the sun via chlorophyll, a pigment that absorbs light. It is packed with powerful nutrients, minerals, and fatty acids, and adding it to your daily ritual creates an alkaline environment in the body. A cup of chlorophyll a day will keep body odor and inflammation at bay.

reishi mother

relieves stress and promotes longevity

Put yourself in the arms of the ultimate healer reishi, one of the most revered and beneficial mushrooms in existence. Reishi is nature's gift for stress management and is an ideal adaptogen to have on hand in your home. This delicate elixir can be supercharged by adding in other adaptogens like ashwaganda, cordyceps, astragalus, or Fo-Ti, and is best for days when self-love and spiritual nourishment are needed.

At the end of your day, pour this elixir into your sacred cup, and sip like a dessert to encourage centeredness and inner strength.

makes 2 cups ||| takes 15 minutes ||| best consumed immediately

ingredients

||| 5 pitted dates
||| ¾ cup water
||| 1 teaspoon fresh lemon juice
||| 1 teaspoon reishi powder (use fruiting body extract when possible)
||| 1 teaspoon vanilla extract
||| ⅛ teaspoon ground Ceylon cinnamon
||| Himalayan salt
||| 1 cup ice
||| cayenne, for garnish (optional)

special tools

||| blender

1. Soak the dates in warm water until soft, then drain and set aside.
2. In a blender, combine the soaked dates, water, lemon juice, reishi, vanilla, cinnamon, and a pinch of salt. Blend until creamy and smooth, about 3 minutes.
3. Add the ice to the blender and blend until crushed.
4. Pour into a glass and garnish with a sprinkle of cayenne (if using) before serving.

reishi   mushroom of spiritual potency

One of the best-known and well-studied adaptogens, reishi has such profound benefits that some consider it a panacea, even calling it the "elixir of immortality." It is rich with the antioxidant beta glucan, the most powerful immune-protecting substance. An essential ingredient in Chinese medicine, it is used to boost the immune system, relieve stress, and promote longevity. Taking reishi encourages a sense of balance, calm, and inner strength.

licorice ticklish

adrenal love

I turn to this recipe when I know I am in a state of fatigue and adrenal burnout. Like many, I lead a fast-paced life and pay the price for it. There are days when I feel like I'm being chased by an imaginary tiger, and the fall seems imminent. On those days, I turn to this elixir for adrenal support, sipping it slowly, taking a moment to recharge.

Drink this like an afternoon cocktail—pour it over ice and sip outdoors among lush greenery. Or imagine yourself sitting on a sun-warmed patio on a summer day.

Health tip: Do not take in high doses if you have high blood pressure or are pregnant.

makes 3 cups ||| takes 15 minutes ||| best consumed immediately

ingredients

||| 2 cups water
||| 1 teaspoon licorice root
||| juice of 1 orange
||| 1 teaspoon Bulgarian rose water
||| 1 cup ice, for serving

special tools

||| blender

1. In a medium saucepan, bring the water to a boil and add the licorice root. Remove from heat and let steep, covered, for 10 minutes.
2. Using a strainer, strain out the licorice, then pour the liquid into a blender and add the orange juice and rose water.
3. Blend until frothy and serve over ice.

licorice the sweet root

One of the most valuable of all herbs, licorice is a powerful anti-inflammatory, similar to hydrocortisone and other corticosteroids that help relieve inflammation ranging from arthritis to canker sores. Licorice stimulates the adrenal glands and also reduces the breakdown of steroids by the liver and kidneys. It has been known to help with conditions where the adrenal glands aren't functioning properly, like Addison's disease.

shilajit life

supports holistic endurance

The star of this elixir is a superfood resin that could be the foundation of this entire book. A microdose of the nutrient-dense shilajit can be added to any recipe in this book and has the ability to improve the general condition of just about everything—skin, brain, digestion, sleep, and mood. I have found it to be one of the best carriers of energy in the body. If you want to choose one ingredient in this book to invest in, choose shilajit.

Consume this drink in the morning on an empty stomach. Continue taking daily for 2 to 4 weeks, then take a 6-week break. Repeat. If you notice any digestive discomfort, reduce the amount of shilajit and take with food. Less is more here.

makes 1 cup ||| takes 2 minutes ||| best consumed immediately

ingredients

||| 1 pea-size piece shilajit resin
||| 1 cup water or fresh juice or coconut water
||| ½ teaspoon fresh lemon juice, or to taste (optional)

1. Dissolve the shilajit in the water or fresh juice or coconut water, and add the lemon juice (if using).

shilajit black plant gold

Shilajit is a viscous resin found in the rocks of the Himalayas, that has developed over centuries from slow plant decomposition. It's commonly used in Ayurvedic medicine as an effective and safe supplement to facilitate the movement of mineral deposits to the blood, improve the metabolic processes, and strengthen the overall condition of the body. Fulvic acid and humic acid, which are responsible for energy production in our cells, are found in abundance in shilajit.

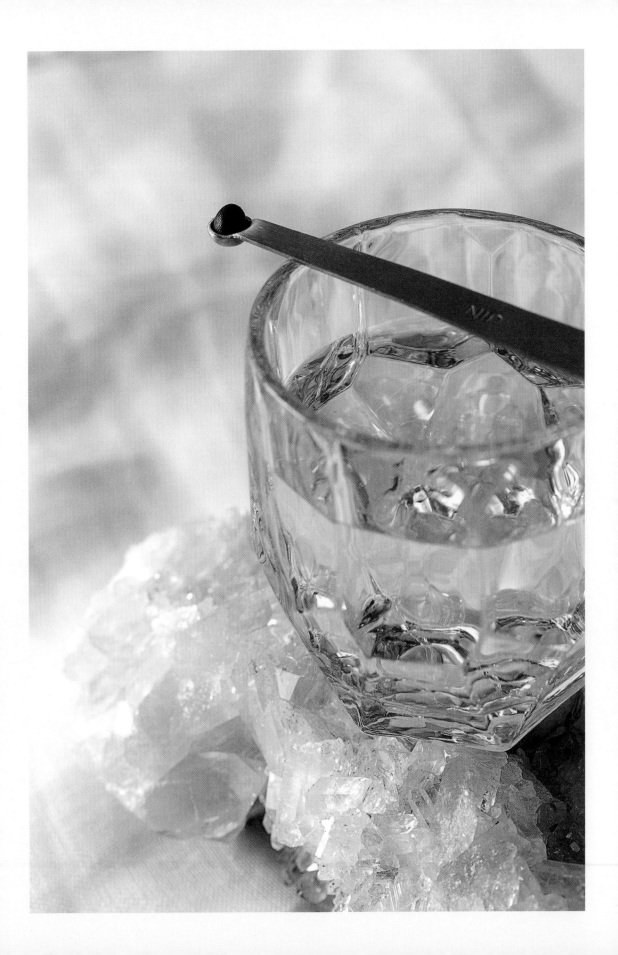

chapter five

cleansing starts on
a cellular level

detox

flush away the toxins

Detoxification means helping your cells get rid of toxins that have accumulated. When your cells are properly hydrated, they can get rid of what they don't need and cleanse themselves through reverse osmosis. Plant elixirs support and tonify the organs so they can complete their detox process, while hydration helps the removal of toxins and flushing of the body through natural processes like sweating, urination, and digestion.

Whether you're looking for a spring cleanse, support for your liver, or recovery from a big night out, return to optimal organ function by choosing one of these plant-based elixirs, and witness the beneficial effects on every system of the body.

blue-green algae lemonade

boosts nutrients and relieves hangovers

Give your body the incredible benefits of one of the original sources of life on Earth. Blue-green algae is rich in protein beta-carotene, and other vital nutrients your body needs to repair and restore itself. There are various types of algae powders—choose chlorella if your body runs cold, and spirulina if your body runs hot.

     Take this as your last drink of the night, or as a "hair of the dog" treatment in the morning, to fuel your body's natural detoxification process.

     Health tip: Not recommended during pregnancy.

makes 1½ cups ||| takes 5 minutes ||| lasts 1 day in the refrigerator

ingredients

||| 1 cup water
||| juice of ½ lemon
||| 1 teaspoon apple cider vinegar
||| 2 teaspoons maple syrup, plus more to taste
||| ⅛ to ¼ teaspoon blue-green algae powder
    (chlorella or spirulina)
||| ½ cup ice, for serving
||| sprigs of mint or basil, for garnish

special tools

||| blender

1. In a blender, combine the water, lemon juice, vinegar, maple syrup, and blue-green algae powder, and blend on high for 1 minute.
2. To serve, pour over ice and garnish with lots of mint or basil.

note: Some algae can have a slight scent, so I like to be generous with the garnishes that will provide a fresh, herbal aroma.

blue-green algae the beginnings of life

Blue-green algae existed before any other plant life. This superfood comes in different forms, including chlorella (a plant) and spirulina (a bacteria). Consumed as a food and a medicine, it is packed with over 65 vitamins, minerals, and enzymes that are easily absorbed by our bodies, making it the perfect source of vitality. There are many wellness benefits to taking blue-green algae, including protection against free radicals, support from bioactives like plant sterols, and the prevention of metabolic and inflammatory diseases.

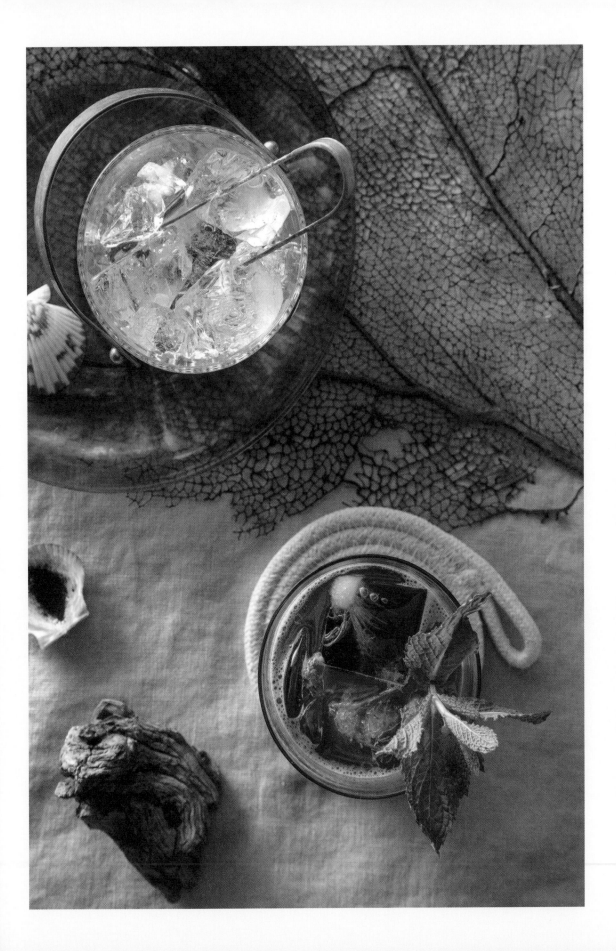

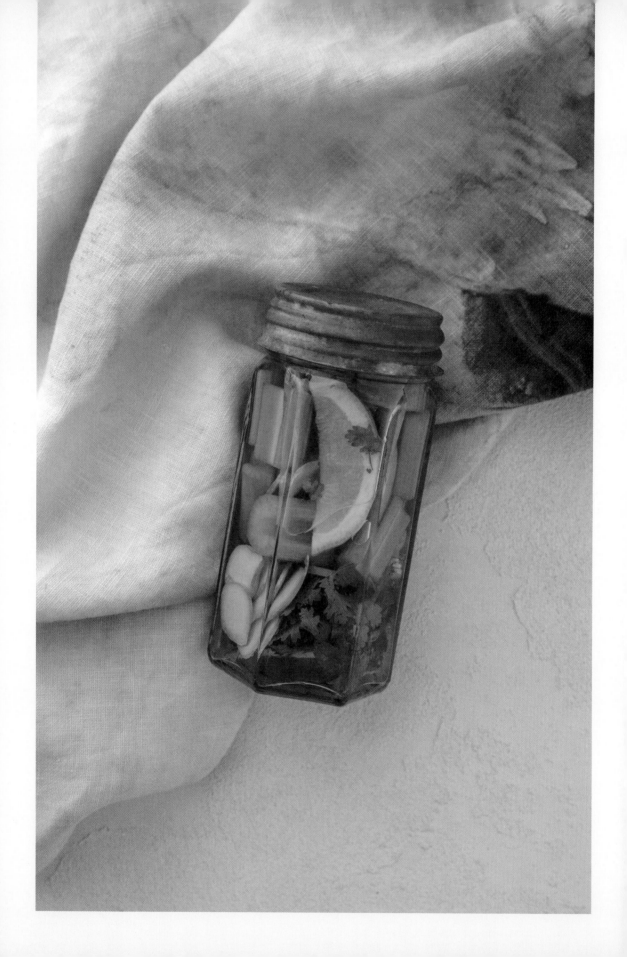

cilantro mercury detox

mineralizes and detoxes from mercury

Why benefit from one green detox machine when you can benefit from two? The combination of celery and cilantro doubles down on the cleansing by supporting the liver, protecting the kidneys, and optimizing the waste-removal process. Sip this savory elixir when your body is calling for a rejuvenating reset and removal.

Sip it all day, every day, as a way to recover from the toxic load that accumulates by interacting with our everyday environment, or if you are a seafood lover in need of a mercury detox.

makes 4 cups ||| takes 5 minutes ||| rests 3 to 24 hours ||| lasts 4 days in the refrigerator

ingredients

||| 1 cup torn cilantro
||| ½ cup parsley
||| 1 (1-inch) piece ginger root, thinly sliced
||| 1 cup celery, roughly chopped
||| juice and rind of ¼ lemon
||| 4 cups water

special tools

||| quart-size jar with airtight lid

1. In a quart-size jar, layer all the ingredients starting with the cilantro, then fill the jar with the water.
2. Seal the jar and let sit in the refrigerator anywhere from 3 to 24 hours before serving.
3. When ready to serve, pour the liquid into a glass, leaving the solid ingredients in the jar.

cilantro the green cleanser

Sometimes called coriander, cilantro is incredibly effective at helping the body reduce its toxic load of heavy metals like mercury, lead, and aluminum. For most, the taste of cilantro is pleasantly tart and citrusy. A small percentage of people are genetically predisposed to detecting the aldehyde chemicals present in cilantro, which turn the taste from a refreshing lemon-lime to the flavor of soap.

moringa spritzer

regenerates the liver

Our liver is constantly at work, quietly filtering our body of what isn't serving us. The proper functioning of this vital organ is critical to our overall health and it deserves to be restored and celebrated. Both moringa and chlorophyll are potent green superfoods that give your body the minerals and nutrients it needs to function. Give a toast to your liver with a sparkling lemonade that will keep you thriving. For greatest enjoyment, make sure the water is very sparkly.

Sip this elixir daily for 4 weeks when you're seeking detoxification, or one to two times a day while breastfeeding to aid milk production.

makes 2 cups ||| takes 10 minutes ||| rests 5 minutes ||| best consumed immediately

ingredients

||| ¼ teaspoon moringa powder
||| 1 teaspoon liquid chlorophyll
||| 3 tablespoons fresh lemon juice
||| 2 cups sparkling water
||| 1 tablespoon maple syrup, plus more to taste
||| ¼ cup mint leaves (about 2 sprigs)
||| ½ cup ice, for serving

special tools

||| matcha whisk
||| quart-size jar with airtight lid
||| muddler

1. In a small bowl, combine the moringa powder, chlorophyll, and lemon juice.
2. Add in a small amount of the sparkling water, then use a matcha whisk to emulsify the ingredients until smooth. (Wash the whisk immediately after using to avoid staining.)
3. Pour the remaining sparkling water into a quart-size jar, then add the contents of the small bowl.
4. Add the maple syrup and mix gently.
5. Using a muddler, muddle a few mint leaves in the bottom of a glass, then pour in the drink and add the ice. Garnish the top with more mint leaves.
6. Chill in the refrigerator for 5 minutes before serving.

moringa   mother's milk

Moringa is so full of health benefits that it is often called "the miracle tree." The leaves are rich in amino acids and tons of highly bioavailable nutrients, minerals, and vitamins. A primary source of nourishment in many countries, moringa is celebrated for everything from increasing milk production in nursing mothers to restoring a damaged liver, which, in turn, supports detoxification, fat metabolizing, and access to nutrients.

burdock and dandelion creamer

spring cleanser and protector

Dandelion root is a key detoxifying herb that works its magic on our bodies by stimulating the liver and gallbladder to clear away waste. I love to drink this herbal elixir when the dandelion starts coming out of the ground, since this is the time of year when our liver is the strongest and most able to handle a detox process.

Sip 1 cup 3 to 4 days a week in the spring while inviting in the new and letting go of the old.

makes 4 cups ||| takes 35 minutes ||| lasts 1 day in the refrigerator

ingredients

||| 1 tablespoon dandelion root
||| 1 tablespoon burdock root
||| 4 cups water
||| 1 tablespoon coconut butter

special tools

||| blender

1. In a medium saucepan, combine the dandelion, burdock, and water.
2. Bring to a boil and simmer for 25 minutes. Let cool.
3. Pour into a blender, add the coconut butter, and blend until creamy.
4. Serve warm or cold. If storing in the refrigerator, blend again before serving to recombine the coconut butter.

dandelion a springtime detoxer

Often dismissed as a weed, this hardy plant can grow in the unlikeliest of places and has unexpected benefits for our health. Sometimes taken as a diuretic to support lowered blood pressure, dandelion also works as a prebiotic, encouraging positive gut flora. Early studies are showing that this antioxidant-rich plant can protect liver tissue when the body is under stress, or toxin levels are high.

chapter six

create an oasis of health inside your body

immunity

self-care before sick care

Helping the body fight disease starts well before we are sick. Our immune system is our first ally against illness, flowing through our body in the form of balance, resistance, and support. Proper hydration allows all of our cells to reach optimal performance and supports their ability to remove waste, carry oxygen, deliver nutrients, and keep tissues healthy.

Take charge of your health by supporting your body during seasonal changes, when it is struggling to keep up with the demands from the environment. Using these elixirs, you can incrementally support your immune system, which is the best way to develop a ritual and a life of self-care.

sage
soother

relieves sore throat

I always find relief from a sore throat by turning to this herbal elixir. If you are prone to a rough, scratchy throat, add this to your daily ritual to stay well throughout the cold season. Sage has antiseptic, antibacterial, and astringent qualities, and has been used for years in the treatment of inflammation of the mouth and throat.

At the first sign of a sore throat, take a 1-ounce shot for immediate, soothing relief. For daily support of the respiratory system and throat, add 1 to 2 tablespoons of this elixir to 1 cup of water and sip during the day. Or make nature's perfect lozenges by adding a larger amount of honey and coconut oil and freezing the elixir in an ice tray.

Health tip: Do not consume large doses during pregnancy.

makes 2 cups ||| takes 50 minutes ||| lasts 7 days in the refrigerator

ingredients

||| 3 cups water
||| 10 leaves fresh sage or ⅓ cup dried sage
||| cayenne
||| 2 tablespoons raw honey, plus more to taste
||| juice of 1 lemon

special tools

||| quart-size jar with airtight lid

1. In a medium saucepan, combine the water, sage, and a pinch of cayenne.
2. Bring to a boil, then simmer with a lid off until the liquid reduces by about one third (about 45 minutes).
3. Using a strainer, strain out the solid ingredients, then pour the liquid into a quart-size jar.
4. Add the honey and lemon juice and stir.
5. Drink warm, or store in the refrigerator until ready to serve. Warm before serving.

sage the sacred ceremonial protector

From cleansing a space to soothing a sore throat, improving digestion, and encouraging regular moon cycles, aromatic sage is there for you. The medieval saying "Why should a man die while sage grows in his garden?" highlights the diverse benefits of this low-growing, fuzzy-leaved shrub. Many indigenous cultures of the Americas have used sage for cleansing spaces through smudging, or by burning small amounts to create an atmosphere of spiritual purification.

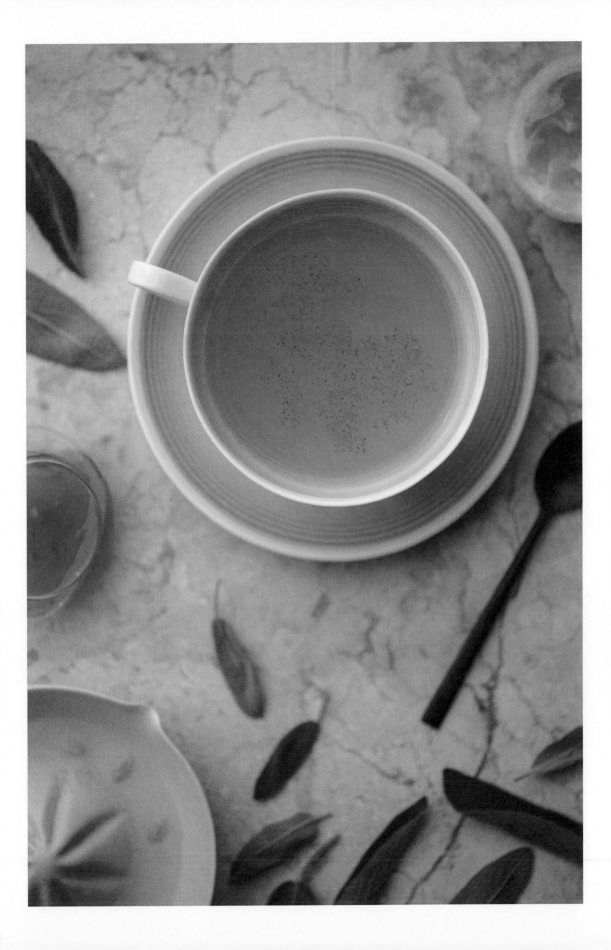

astragalus broth

pre-cold-and-flu helper

An elevated (and plant-based) version of my dad's bone broth. Just like his, this warming savory elixir is designed to increase your immune system reserves so that you can protect against seasonal maladies like cold and flu.

In the winter, simmer a pot of this recipe often and sip a cup or two several times a week to stay strong and healthy.

Health tip: Not recommended for those taking medications for the immune system or with acute illnesses.

makes 4 cups ||| takes about 3 hours ||| lasts 5 days in the refrigerator

ingredients

||| 1 tablespoon coconut oil
||| 2 to 3 stalks celery, cut into 1-inch pieces
||| ½ parsnip or carrot, cut into 1-inch pieces
||| ½ large red or white onion, quartered
||| 7 to 10 cloves garlic, peeled
||| 2 sprigs thyme
||| 2 sprigs rosemary
||| ⅓ cup fresh dill, chopped
||| 5 cups water

||| 1 tablespoon astragalus bark
||| 1 teaspoon medicinal mushrooms, such as reishi, chaga, lion's mane, or turkey tail (optional)
||| salt and pepper

special tools

||| quart-size jar with airtight lid

1. In a large saucepan, heat the coconut oil over medium heat.
2. Once the oil is shimmering, add the celery, parsnip or carrot, and onion, and sauté for 3 minutes or until fragrant.
3. Add the garlic, thyme, rosemary, and dill, and sauté until the garlic is golden, lowering the heat if needed to avoid burning.
4. Add the water, astragalus, and medicinal mushrooms (if using) to the saucepan. Bring to a boil, then cover and simmer on low heat for 2 to 3 hours.
5. Using a strainer, strain out the solid ingredients, and pour the liquid into a quart-size jar, then add the garlic back in for increased potency.
6. Season with salt and pepper.
7. Sip warm, or store in the refrigerator in an airtight jar until ready to serve.

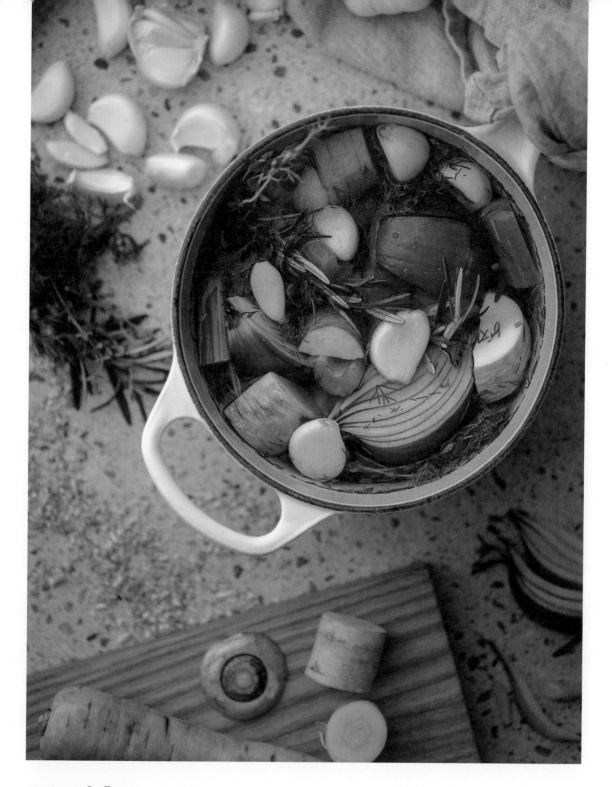

astragalus breathe, for life

Sometimes called the most powerful immune-boosting adaptogen on Earth, astragalus has been an important component of Chinese medicine for thousands of years. It is thought to strengthen the lungs and qi energy and prevent against illness by fortifying the immune system. It is loaded with polysaccharides, which help encourage the activity of T-cells, the antibodies created by our immune system.

winter fire cider

fights cold and flu

This is my version of a recipe used in many cultures, which combines vinegar, spices, and garlic. In the 1960s, when herbalist Rosemary Gladstar helped popularize traditional medicine in the United States, she gave this elixir the name "fire cider."

Tap into ancient wisdom by preparing this elixir in the fall and consuming it throughout the flu season. For prevention, add 1 to 2 tablespoons to warm or tepid water and sip daily. For treatment, take a 1-ounce shot at the first sign of symptoms.

makes 4 cups concentrate (about 40 to 60 servings) ||| takes 10 minutes ||| rests 3 to 4 weeks ||| lasts 6 months at room temperature

ingredients

- 4 cups apple cider vinegar
- 1 (4-inch) piece ginger root, grated
- 1 (4-inch) piece turmeric root, grated
- juice and peel of 1 lemon
- juice and peel of 1 orange
- 1 tablespoon Ceylon cinnamon bark or 1 stick broken into chunks
- 4 cloves garlic, chopped
- 3 tablespoons dried Schisandra berries
- 1 tablespoon adaptogen of choice, such as reishi, ashwagandha, or astragalus (optional)
- 4 tablespoons maple syrup
- 2 tablespoons cayenne
- black pepper

special tools

- quart-size jar with airtight lid

1. In a medium saucepan, warm the vinegar over low heat.
2. In a quart-size jar, combine the ginger, turmeric, juice and peel of lemon and orange, cinnamon, garlic, Schisandra berries, and your adaptogen of choice (if using), then add the warmed vinegar. Seal with a lid.
3. Place the jar in a warm spot near a sunny window and let sit for 3 to 4 weeks, shaking occasionally.
4. When ready to drink, strain out the solid ingredients using a strainer, and return the liquid to the jar. Add the maple syrup, cayenne, and a pinch of black pepper.
5. Store up to 6 months in a dark place at room temperature.

garlic an understated hero

We know garlic as a pungent culinary ingredient, but less known is its incredible antioxidant, antimicrobial, antiviral, and antibiotic nature. It is also thought to act as a decongestant and expectorant, making it nature's ideal cold and flu remedy. Some studies point to the sulfur in garlic as the component that helps improve our health.

chamomile chia boost

pictured on page 78

battles seasonal allergies

An overloaded immune system is often closely tied to inflammation in the body and poor digestive health. This gentle elixir helps take your body out of fight mode, so your immune system can do its job with ease. Soothing, calming German chamomile is an accessible, simple herbal medicine that I recommend as a staple herb for everyone's medicine cabinet.

Sip this drink all day long when you're feeling run down, and during allergy season to keep your immune system charged.

makes 4 cups ||| takes 15 minutes ||| rests overnight ||| lasts 4 days in the refrigerator

ingredients

||| 4 cups water
||| 1 tablespoon dried German chamomile
||| 1 pear, quartered
||| 1 (2-inch) piece ginger root, sliced
||| 2 Ceylon cinnamon sticks
||| 1 vanilla bean, split and seeds scraped
||| 1 teaspoon chia seeds

special tools

||| quart-size jar with airtight lid

1. In a medium saucepan, bring the water to a boil.
2. Add the chamomile, and let steep for 10 minutes.
3. Using a strainer, strain out the chamomile, then pour the liquid into a quart-size jar. Add the pear, ginger, cinnamon, seeds and pod of the vanilla bean, and chia seeds.
4. Seal the jar with a lid and shake for 1 minute to mix, then let sit overnight.
5. When ready to serve, shake well, as the chia seeds will rise to the top. Pour the liquid into a glass, leaving the solid ingredients in the jar.

Chamomile **nature's sleep aid**

Chamomile's healing benefits don't stop at digestion (page 27). It is also known for its powerful ability to soothe and relax. Dried and steeped into a tea, this apple-scented herb has anti-inflammatory and antispasmodic properties and can relieve nervous tension and irritability, which makes it an ideal addition to your bedtime rituals.

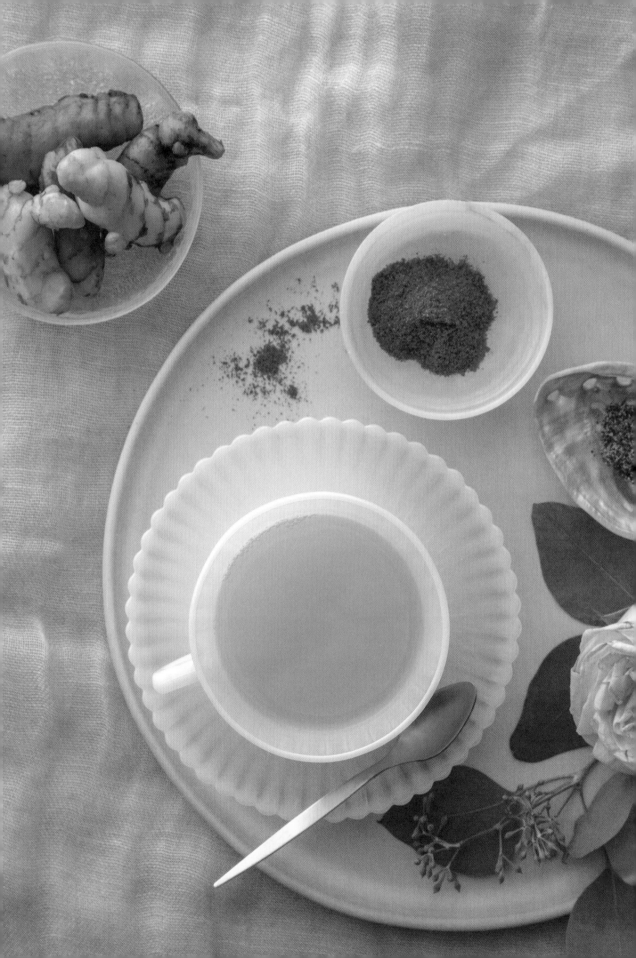

turmeric booster

maintains immune system

Inflammation is the fertile soil that allows dis-ease to grow. The unparalleled anti-inflammatory benefits of turmeric make it the perfect ingredient for a daily immunity elixir. I developed this as an accessible and enjoyable way to help you prevent flu and colds, all season long. A word to the wise: Turmeric will stain your hands and kitchen. When working with the fresh root, take care to prevent contact with skin, fabrics, and countertops.

Sip 1 cup every day in the afternoon to help your body recover from injury or exercise, and to protect against seasonal illness. Or use it for prevention and make turmeric water by adding 1 ounce of the elixir to 1 cup of water.

makes 4 cups ||| takes 20 minutes ||| lasts 3 days in the refrigerator

ingredients

||| 4 cups water
||| 1 (2-inch) piece turmeric root, grated
||| cayenne
||| black pepper
||| ⅓ cup fresh orange juice
||| juice of ½ lemon
||| 1 teaspoon apple cider vinegar
||| 1 tablespoon raw honey, plus more to taste

special tools

||| quart-size jar with airtight lid

1. In a medium saucepan, combine the water, turmeric, a pinch of cayenne, and a pinch of black pepper, and bring to a boil.
2. Simmer for 15 minutes, then strain out the solid ingredients using a strainer, and pour the liquid into a quart-size jar.
3. Add the orange juice, lemon juice, vinegar, and honey to the jar and stir. Seal with a lid and store in the refrigerator.
4. Warm before serving.

turmeric the golden spice

A root related to ginger, bright yellow turmeric is a familiar addition to curries, and is also an important element of Ayurvedic medicine. The active ingredient curcumin is believed to relieve inflammation in the body and support digestion, which is the foundation of good health. Turmeric is used to balance blood sugar, lower cholesterol, and prevent seasonal colds and flus.

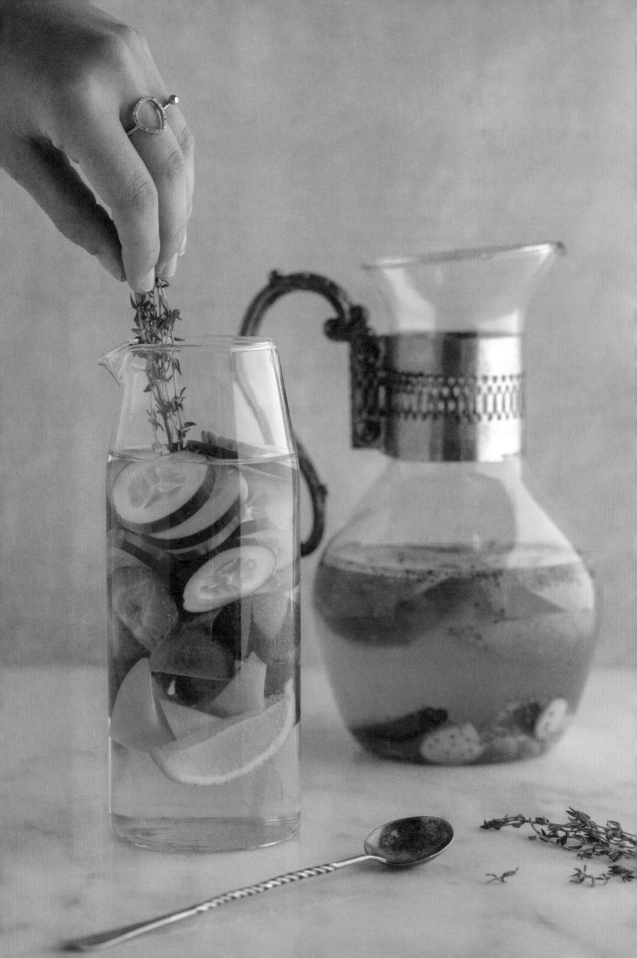

thyme
life

supports respiration

Thyme, nature's respiratory system aid, has powerful antiseptic properties that make it a useful addition in this immunity elixir. Easily grown and widely available, this herb can help clear the lungs of congestion, calm coughing, and help you heal and breathe more easily. I've used my favorite antioxidant-rich berries in this recipe, but you can use any that are fresh and in season.

If you are prone to respiratory challenges, add this elixir to your daily rituals in the seasons when berries are at their peak.

makes 4 cups ||| takes 5 minutes ||| rests 3 to 24 hours ||| lasts 3 days in the refrigerator

ingredients

||| ¼ lemon, cut into wedges
||| ½ cup cherries, pitted
||| ½ cup strawberries, cut in half
||| ½ English cucumber, sliced
||| 2 small bunches fresh thyme (enough
    to fill ¼ of the jar)
||| 4 cups water

special tools

||| quart-size jar with airtight lid

1. In a quart-size jar, layer all the ingredients starting with the lemon, then fill the jar with the water (for a more intense flavor, boil the water first).
2. Seal the jar and let sit in the refrigerator anywhere from 3 to 24 hours before serving.
3. When ready to serve, pour the liquid into a glass, leaving the solid ingredients in the jar.

thyme the original antiseptic

A popular herb in cooking, thyme is becoming more widely known for its incredible antiseptic and antibacterial properties. Thyme works to heal any infection, whether bacterial or viral. The ancient Egyptians used thyme in their embalming rituals, but more recently, it is used to relieve stomach ulcers, hay fever, and asthma, and to soothe the nerves.

chapter seven

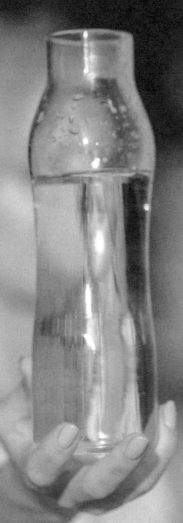

nourishing your mind is
nourishing your creativity

brainpower

pause and absorb

Supporting your brain is supporting the complex engine that allows you to engage with the world around you. Your brain knows you are drinking liquid even before your body has absorbed what you've taken in. It then takes 10 to 15 minutes for the water to be absorbed and you are truly rehydrated. Support your brain by creating a habit of sipping water throughout the day, putting your body in a perpetual state of absorption and your brain at ease knowing your hydration levels are sufficient. By enhancing your water with powerful ingredients, you can use this daily ritual to support memory, regenerate brain health, and increase mental stamina.

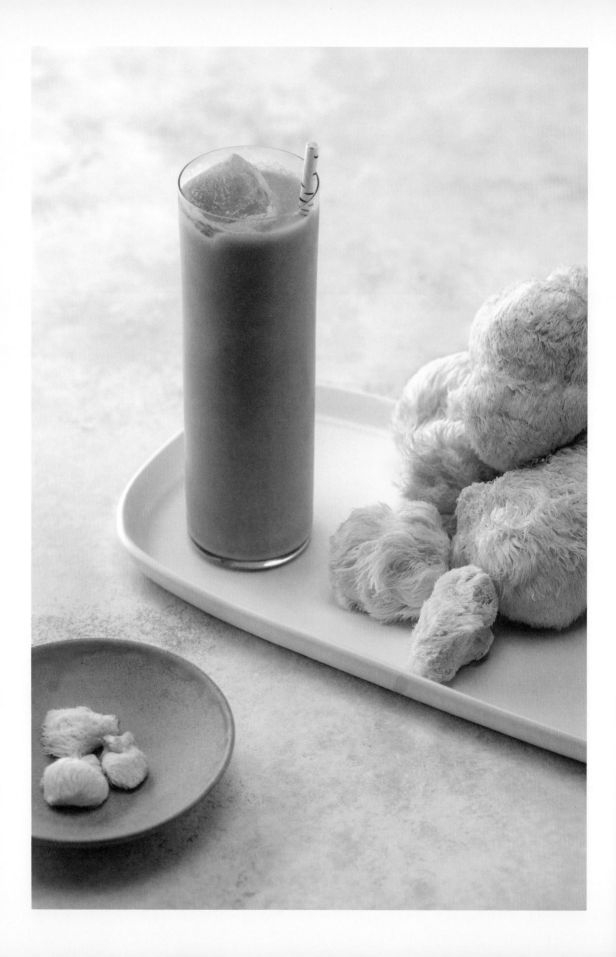

lion's mane matcha

regenerates the brain

Use this elixir to help protect against brain degeneration that can naturally occur as we age. The moderate caffeine in matcha will keep you going in the moment, and the lion's mane will keep you sharp in the long run.

Make this drink when you are entering a period of stress—this is when our system gets depleted the most. Sipping in the morning or early afternoon is best, as this elixir is quite energizing.

makes 2 cups ||| takes 5 minutes ||| best consumed immediately

ingredients

||| 1 teaspoon matcha
||| ½ teaspoon lion's mane powder
||| 2 tablespoons coconut butter
||| ½ teaspoon vanilla extract
||| 1 tablespoon raw honey
||| 1¼ cups water
||| ½ cup ice, for serving

special tools

||| blender

1. In a blender, combine the matcha, lion's mane, coconut butter, vanilla, honey, and water.
2. Blend for 1 minute or until the coconut butter is emulsified and the elixir is creamy.
3. Pour the elixir over ice and let rest for 1 minute until chilled.

note: Make sure the coconut butter is mixed well before using in this recipe, as the texture of the drink could otherwise become gritty.

lion's mane a mushroom like no other

Lion's mane looks like nothing else on the forest floor, making it one of the safest mushrooms to forage. It contains special compounds that have been known to stimulate the growth and maintenance of brain cells and has been used as a brain-health supplement for years. Some early studies have shown that lion's mane may be effective in the treatment of Alzheimer's, which is characterized by a degeneration of brain cells.

gotu kola
alert

fortifies mental stamina and working memory

I use this to keep my brain fully charged and offer this to my team before meetings. Designed to increase your mental capacity to the fullest, this elixir helps you access as much of your working memory as possible.

You can prepare this recipe several times a week before bed, and wake up to a cup of brain health. Take a 1-ounce shot daily or add to 1 cup of water to dilute. This elixir is good for those starting to sense their memory declining with age.

makes 4 cups ||| takes 5 minutes ||| rests overnight ||| lasts 1 day

ingredients

||| 4 cups water
||| 2 tablespoons fresh mint or peppermint or spearmint, or 1 tablespoon dried
||| 1 tablespoon dried ginkgo
||| 1 small sprig rosemary, finely chopped, or 1 tablespoon dried
||| 1 tablespoon dried gotu kola
||| fresh lemon juice to taste

special tools

||| quart-size jar with airtight lid

1. Bring the water to a boil.
2. In a quart-size jar, layer all the ingredients, then cover with the boiling water.
3. Seal the jar and let sit in the refrigerator overnight.
4. When ready to serve, strain out the herbs and return the liquid to the jar.

gotu kola herb of longevity

In herbal medicine this revitalizing herb is used topically and in elixirs. Ayurvedic tradition believes gotu kola is beneficial for treating skin conditions, supporting a healthy nervous system, and relieving anxiety. Gotu kola is also known to increase cognitive capacity by improving consistent blood delivery to the brain, repairing mucus membranes, and supporting communication between the gut and the brain.

remembering rosemary with CBD oil

pictured on pages 86–87

supports memory and concentration

Rosemary is one of my top herbs to use for overall health, which starts with the brain. If you're asking yourself whether or not your memory could use some support, you probably already know the answer. Rosemary triggers the brain and engages the senses, while CBD will help you concentrate. Take this memory-enhancing elixir, supercharged with CBD oil, to give you the extra help you need and strengthen your long-term memory.

Sip 1 cup three to four times a week when you need extra sharpness and brainpower for studying or working on a big project. While sipping, take a moment to enjoy the aroma of rosemary. Alternatively, you can take the CBD oil sublingually (under the tongue) and wash it down with the elixir.

Health tip: Taking too much CBD oil may cause a drop in blood sugar, so use only the recommended amount.

makes 4 cups ||| takes 50 minutes ||| lasts 4 days in the refrigerator

ingredients

||| 4 cups water
||| 6 to 8 tablespoons fresh rosemary, chopped
||| 6 to 8 tablespoons fresh thyme, chopped
||| 1 tablespoon fresh lemon juice
||| raw honey to taste
||| CBD oil

special tools

||| quart-size jar with airtight lid

1. Bring the water to a boil.
2. Place the rosemary and thyme in a quart-size jar (they should fill ¼ of the jar).
3. Pour the boiling water into the jar, then let steep for 30 to 45 minutes.
4. Using a strainer, strain out the herbs, and return the liquid to the jar.
5. Add the lemon juice and honey.
6. Refrigerate until ready to drink. Before serving, add a dose of CBD oil (as recommended on the bottle) to 1 cup of elixir.

CBD oil blazing the trail

CBD (Cannabidiol) oil is derived from hemp, and is most commonly associated with increasing focus, strengthening retention, reducing pain, and easing anxiety. CBD is non-psychoactive, meaning you won't get high, because it does not contain the chemical THC.

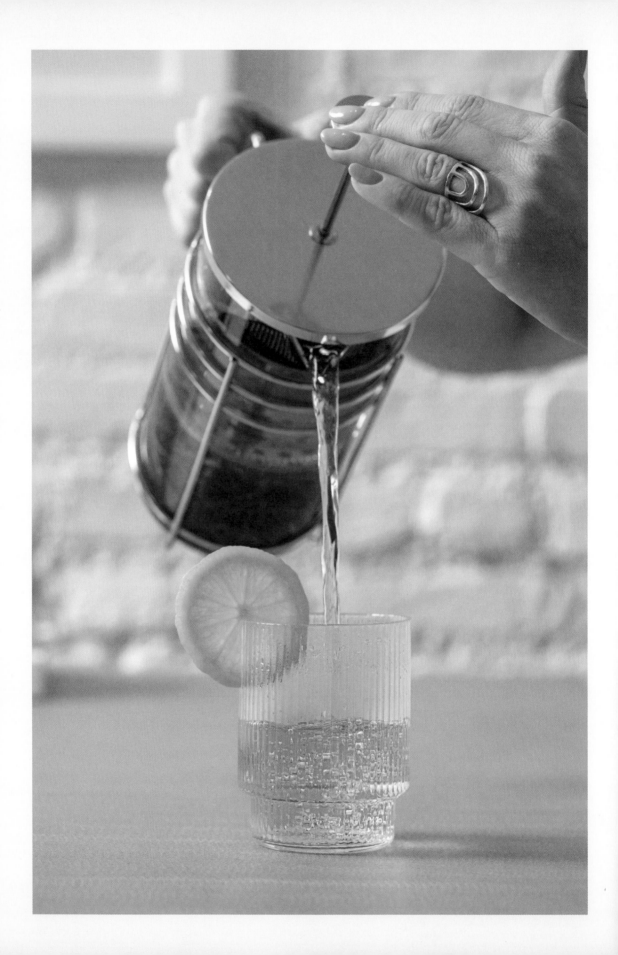

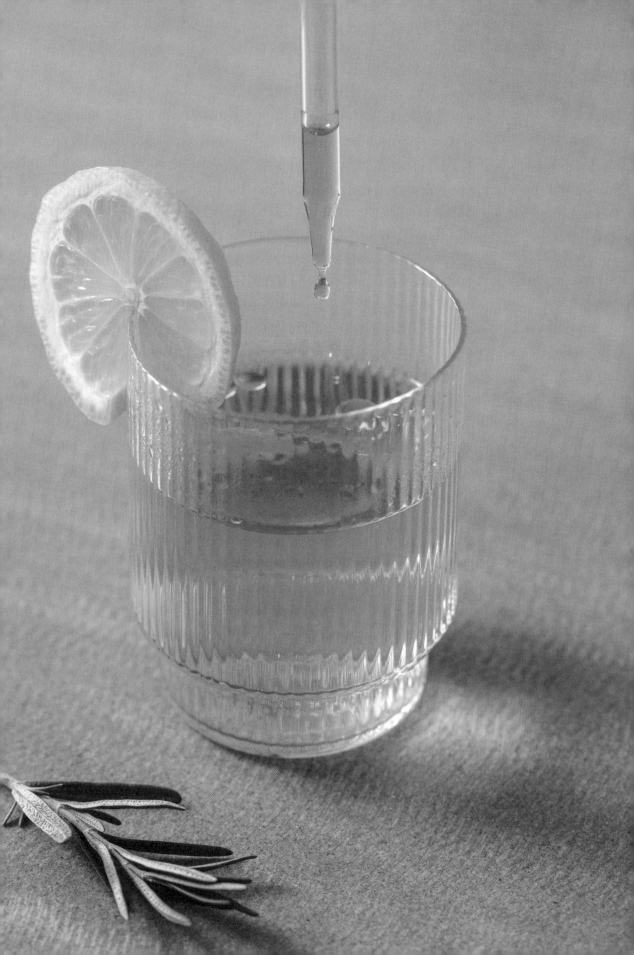

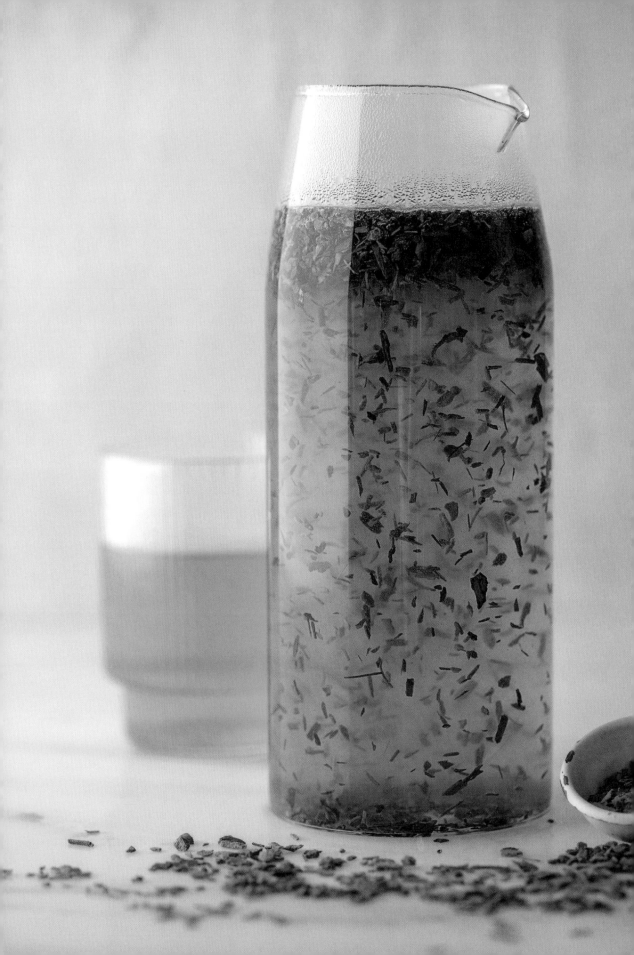

cinnamon flow

invigorates presence and sharpness

Most body types—especially ones that are prone to feeling cold—can benefit from increasing the flow of oxygenated blood through the body and to the brain. I've used this warming and surprisingly effective elixir to support healthy cell and organ function, sharpen focus, and fight off bacterial infections.

Take it as a shot in the morning or add to your water bottle daily, sipping before noon for best results.

Health tip: Not recommended for those with a high body temperature or with low blood sugar.

makes 4 cups ||| takes 45 minutes ||| lasts 7 days in the refrigerator

ingredients

||| 4 cups water
||| 3 tablespoons Ceylon cinnamon chips
||| raw honey to taste

special tools

||| quart-size jar with airtight lid

1. Bring the water to a boil.
2. Place the cinnamon in a quart-size jar and add the boiling water. Seal the jar and let steep for 40 minutes.
3. Using a strainer, strain out the solids and return the liquid to the jar.
4. Add the honey and stir.
5. Refrigerate until ready to drink. Take 1 ounce as a shot in the morning or add to 1 cup warm water.

Ceylon cinnamon a bark with a beneficial bite

Cinnamon is a staple in many homes but what is often in the cupboard is cassia cinnamon. Cassia contains large amounts of coumarin, which is thought to be harmful in large doses. I recommend using Ceylon cinnamon for all the recipes in this book. Cinnamon has antibacterial and antiviral properties, eases digestive problems, balances blood sugar, and increases blood circulation. This is a very warming spice that stimulates the body's internal fires.

chapter eight

when we come from a place of
balance, we can find lasting
sources of energy

energy

reach your true potential

There's no other feeling like the energy of being a child—full of authentic, vibrant vitality. Feeling energized is at the heart of how we experience our time on Earth. The key to creating a vital life is to prevent overtaxing our system. Great energy comes from giving back to your body as much as you are taking in order to achieve alignment. Support your system with these elixirs that will keep your body nourished and hydrated, so that you can become fully awake and fill your wellness cup to overflowing.

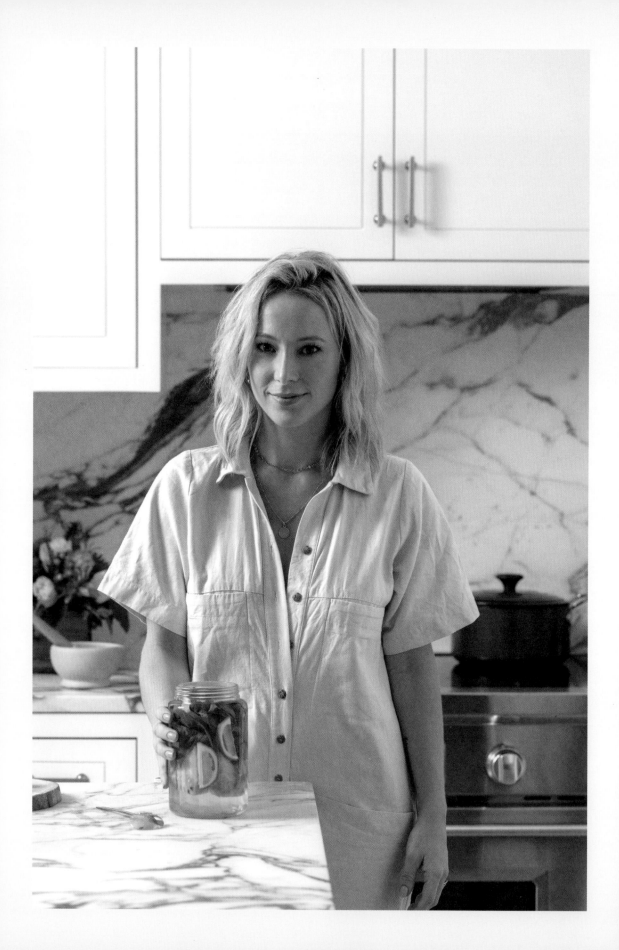

watermelon hydrator

hydrates and provides a magnesium boost

Overcome fatigue by dealing with its root cause: dehydration. Minerals are the foundation of proper hydration, as maintaining them in optimal levels helps with oxygenation throughout the body. Infusing water with the mineral-rich watermelon creates nature's perfect electrolyte balancer. This colorful, fun elixir is a great way to get kids to drink more water, too.

Reach for this recipe in hot and sweaty summer months and turn your love of watermelons into your new go-to energy drink.

makes 4 cups ||| takes 5 minutes ||| rests 3 to 24 hours ||| lasts 2 days in the refrigerator

ingredients

||| 2 cups cubed watermelon
||| juice and rind of ½ lime
||| 20 basil leaves or 2 large sprigs (use variegated basil for a more beautiful elixir)
||| Himalayan salt to taste
||| 4 cups water

special tools

||| quart-size jar with airtight lid

1. In a quart-size jar, layer all the ingredients starting with the watermelon, then fill the jar with the water.
2. Seal the jar and let sit in the refrigerator anywhere from 3 to 24 hours before serving.
3. When ready to serve, pour the liquid into a glass, leaving the solid ingredients in the jar.

watermelon nature's perfect hydrator

Beautiful and hydrating, the watermelon is made up of 90 percent water and is naturally high in electrolytes like potassium and magnesium, which help your body maintain a healthy fluid balance. A member of the melon family, it gets its brilliant red color from high levels of lycopene, a powerful antioxidant also found in tomatoes.

chaga coffee

revitalizes the whole body

This is a favorite recipe of mine. When I was first introduced to chaga, I realized the powerful effects it had on my health, which is why I'm passionate about helping others incorporate this supporter, builder, and energy enhancer into their daily rituals. Chaga is a potent, antioxidizing adaptogen that will give your body the longer-term support it needs, long after the caffeine buzz has worn off. True, lasting energy is a by-product of your body feeling and operating at its best.

In this recipe you'll be making a chaga base, which you can drink on its own as a morning shot of energy, or incorporate into your everyday coffee routine by using it instead of water. Whichever you end up doing, drink the chaga base every morning as your daily defender of vitality and longevity, and tap into energy resources that will have you feeling immortal.

Health tip: Consult your doctor before using if you are taking prescription drugs.

the base: makes about 16 cups ||| takes 3 to 4 hours ||| lasts 15 days in the refrigerator
the elixir: makes 4 cups ||| takes 15 minutes ||| best consumed immediately

ingredients

for the chaga base
||| 2 gallons water
||| ⅓ cup ground chaga or 4 to 5 small chaga rocks

for the coffee
||| 4 tablespoons ground coffee
||| 4 cups chaga base

special tools

||| Large airtight jar or pitcher (that fits 1 to 1½ gallons of liquid)
||| French press

make the chaga base
1. In a large saucepan, bring the water to a boil. Add the chaga, and simmer on low for 3 to 4 hours. The volume may reduce by half, depending on your stove.
2. Using a strainer, strain out the solids, if any, and store in a jar or pitcher in the refrigerator for up to 15 days.

make the coffee
1. Place the ground coffee in a French press (I suggest 1 tablespoon of coffee per cup, but feel free to make coffee to your liking).
2. In a large saucepan, bring the chaga base to a boil, then add to the French press.
3. Let steep for 5 minutes, then press down the filter.

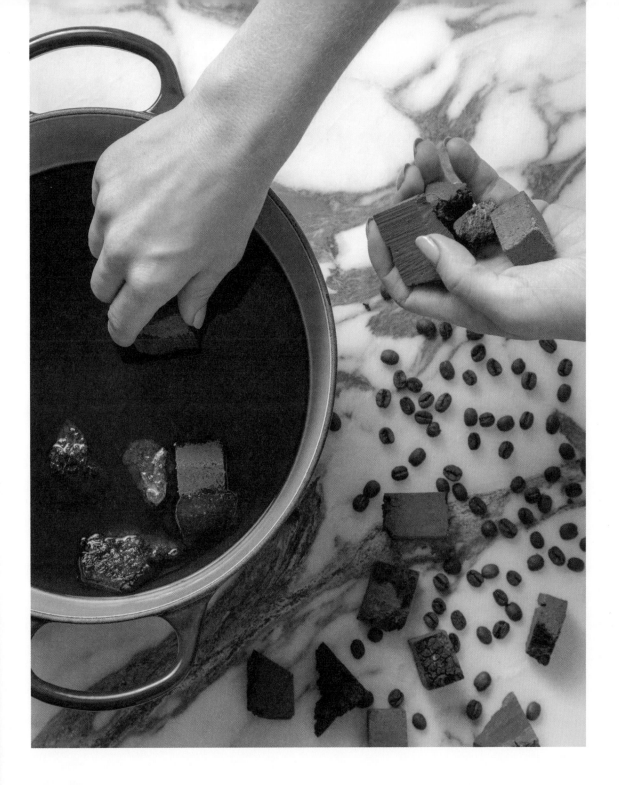

chaga the diamond of the forest

This nutrient-dense adaptogenic mushroom helps boost your immune system during times of sickness, as well as slowing it down if it becomes overactive (autoimmune illnesses). Chaga grows symbiotically on birch trees as a dark, woody mass, and strengthens the host tree by producing phytochemicals to guard against disease. Similarly, our ability to prevent sickness is also increased when we consume phytochemicals.

cordyceps and hazelnut push-up

invigorates and enhances performance

Find pleasure and power in every sip of this warm cocoa-inspired energy elixir. The oxygenating super-adaptogen cordyceps creates a balance between stimulating and supporting your adrenal glands, which in turn gives you more power for physically challenging tasks.

Drink 1 cup 30 minutes before or after a workout to break through hurdles, find your edge, and set some new personal bests, all while avoiding burnout (and sugary energy drinks).

Health tip: Not recommended for those with autoimmune diseases.

makes 2 cups ||| takes 5 minutes ||| best consumed immediately

ingredients

||| 2 teaspoons cordyceps powder
||| 2 tablespoons hazelnut butter or natural chocolate spread
||| ¼ to ½ teaspoon chili powder (depending on potency and preference)
||| Himalayan salt
||| 2 cups water
||| maple syrup to taste

special tools

||| blender

1. In a blender, combine the cordyceps powder, hazelnut butter, chili powder, a pinch of salt, and water, and blend until smooth.
2. Add the maple syrup and serve immediately.

note: For a special treat, make a creamy version by adding 1 tablespoon of tocos or coconut butter before blending.

cordyceps   the mushroom of vitality and vigor

Alongside reishi, cordyceps is considered to be one of the most powerful adaptogenic mushrooms. It grows mainly in tropical forests and was once so rare that it was reserved only for emperors. Cordyceps can be used to create a powerful energy elixir, and it is known to revitalize sex glands and reproductive systems. It also supports recovery from adrenal depletion and increases oxygen utilization.

beet
electrified

pictured on pages 98–99

boosts nitrogen and supports circulation

Inspired by a juice I've been serving to athletes for years, this elixir is designed to supercharge your body and your blood. Beets naturally increase nitric oxide in the blood, and ginkgo increases blood flow—when taken together, they create the perfect performance conditions in the body.

Drink this before a long run, an intense spin class, or any endurance activity for that extra edge. Sip it four to five times a week before a strenuous competition.

Health tip: Do not take ginkgo biloba if you are taking blood-thinning medication.

makes 4 cups ||| takes 30 minutes ||| lasts 2 days in the refrigerator

ingredients

||| 4 cups water
||| ½ cup cubed green apple
||| ½ cup cubed beets
||| 1 tablespoon dried ginkgo biloba
||| juice of ½ lime, or to taste

special tools

||| mortar and pestle
||| French press

1. Bring the water to a boil.
2. Using a mortar and pestle, crush the apples and place in the French press.
3. Add the beets and ginkgo to the French press, then fill with boiling water.
4. Let steep for 20 minutes, then press down the filter.
5. Let rest in the refrigerator, and add the lime juice before serving.

ginkgo biloba fan-shaped support

The ancient ginkgo tree is the only living species of its kind—all others became extinct during the time of the dinosaurs. Its fan-shaped leaves are used in dried form, as well as an extract. Ginkgo's health benefits include maintaining plentiful blood flow to the central nervous system and the brain, and clearing out phlegm which can build up in the respiratory system and prevent the proper oxygenation of the body.

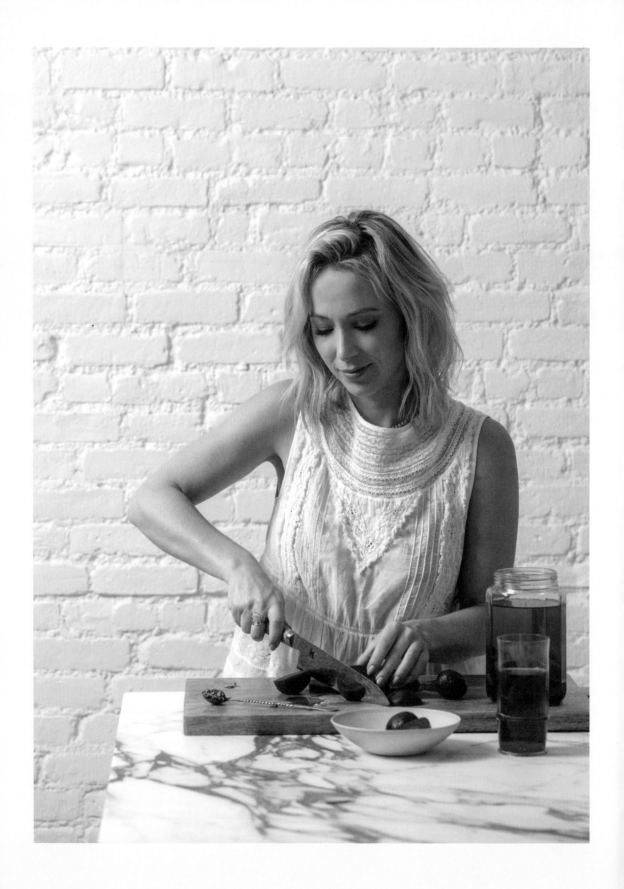

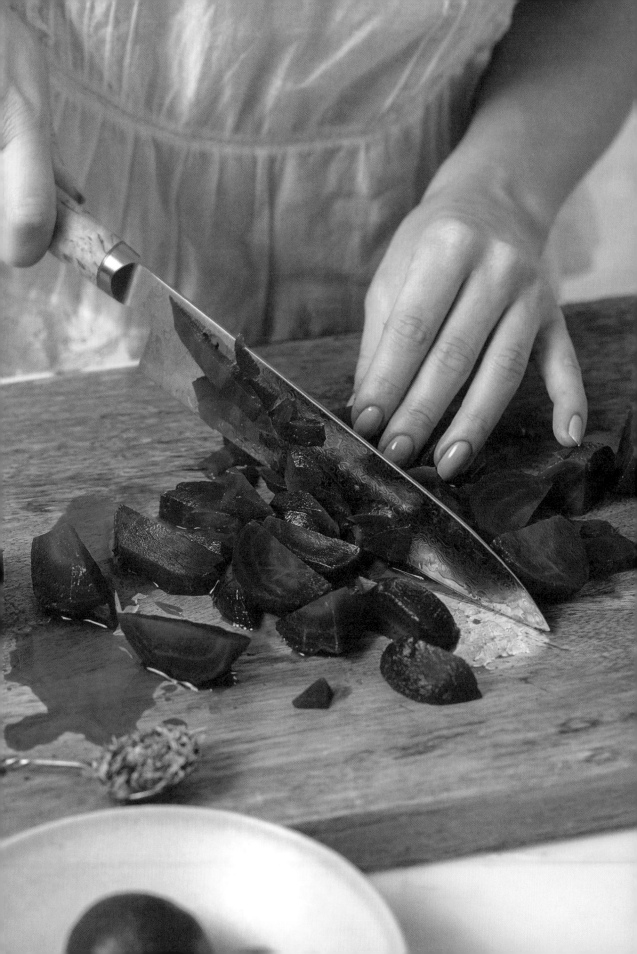

chapter nine

embrace change
to feel balanced

mood

flow toward joy

Wellness is a flow—when we allow our thoughts to flow like water, we can release stagnation and what isn't serving us, and move to a joyful place. The same is true for our bodies. When we are hydrated and nourished, the good (like balance and vitality) is able to flow in, and the bad (like waste and toxins) can flow out. Our mood is a conversation our body is having with us, letting us know when we need to adjust our energy and move toward calmness, vibrancy, joy, or love.

Cultures around the world use beverages like tea, coffee, or cocktails, to boost mood and create a ritual of community. Use this foundation to build a new type of celebration, and toast to nourishing your ability to maintain equilibrium throughout your days.

rhodiola mint chocolate

elevates mood and vitality

When you've been burning the candle at both ends, know you can find support in this elixir. Designed to help the body overcome the effects of long-term stress and boost overall vitality, this fresh-tasting recipe will lift up your mind and body.

At the first signs of stress-related mental exhaustion, create this uplifting drink and sip once a day, especially when you're feeling nervous, exhausted, facing a mild depression, or are on the edge of a burnout.

Health tip: If taken too often, this may cause irritability and sleep disturbances. If you are manic or bipolar, avoid this elixir.

makes 3 cups ||| takes 20 minutes ||| best consumed immediately

ingredients

||| 2 cups water
||| ½ cup fresh mint leaves, plus more
  for garnish
||| 2 tablespoons coconut oil
||| 4 teaspoons cacao powder
||| 1 teaspoon rhodiola powder
||| 2 tablespoons tocos powder
||| 4 teaspoons maple syrup
||| ½ cup ice (optional)
||| shaved raw chocolate, for garnish (optional)

special tools

||| French press
||| blender

1. Bring the water to a boil.
2. Place the mint leaves in a French press and cover with the boiling water. Let steep for 15 minutes, then press down the filter.
3. Using a strainer, strain out the mint, and pour the liquid into a blender. Add the coconut oil, cacao, rhodiola, tocos, and maple syrup, and blend for 45 seconds.
4. Serve immediately for a warm drink, or let it cool, add the ice, and blend for a chilled treat.
5. Garnish generously with mint and shaved raw chocolate (if using) and serve.

note: To make a creamier elixir, reduce the amount of water or use coconut butter instead of coconut oil.

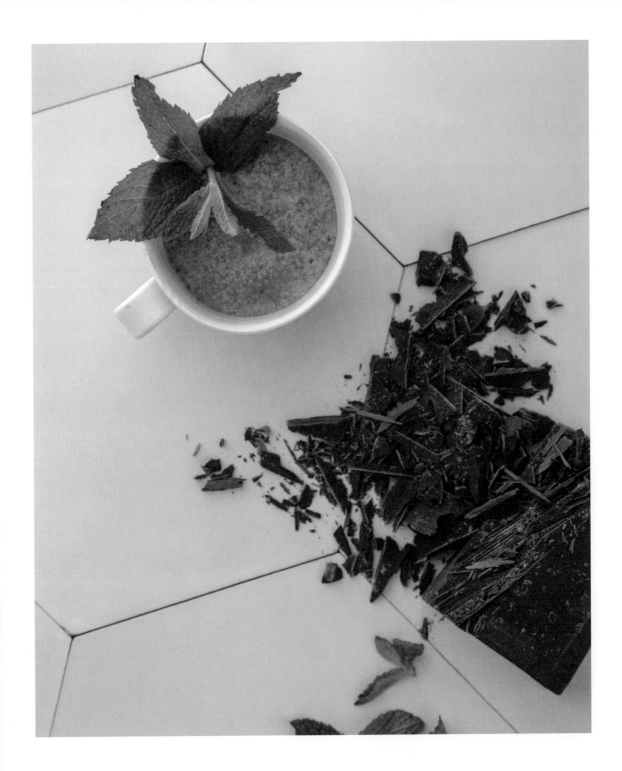

rhodiola rosea arctic gold

Similar to ginseng, rhodiola is the rose-colored root of an Arctic plant that thrives in extreme environments. It has been used for hundreds of years in places like Tibet, Siberia, and Scandinavia to enhance mental performance and promote physical and mental endurance. An anti-inflammatory and an antidepressant, rhodiola is best used for overcoming long-term stress and preventing burnout.

blueberry mood booster

pictured on pages 106–107

captures joyfulness

Some of my happiest memories as a child are of picking blueberries with my grandma on farms in Canada. I knew blueberries created happiness for me then, but I had yet to learn about their high levels of mood-boosting flavonoids, which I came to appreciate later in life. I created this elixir to capture that sense of childhood joy.

Make it in the summertime when blueberries are in season, and drink as often as you need a smile on your face.

makes 4 cups ||| takes 5 minutes ||| rests 3 to 24 hours ||| lasts 3 days in the refrigerator

ingredients

||| juice and rind of ¼ lemon
||| 1 cup blueberries
||| 3 sprigs fresh lavender
||| 1 cup fresh lemon balm, basil, or mint
||| 4 cups water

special tools

||| quart-size jar with airtight lid

1. In a quart-size jar, layer all the ingredients starting with the lemon, then fill the jar with the water.
2. Seal the jar and let sit in the refrigerator anywhere from 3 to 24 hours.
3. When ready to serve, crush the blueberries lightly with a spoon to release extra flavor. Pour the liquid into a glass, leaving the solid ingredients in the jar.

lemon balm the calmer

Related to mint, lemon balm has a noticeably citrusy aroma and is often used to alleviate mild anxiety, sleep problems, and restlessness. A powerful antioxidant and anti-inflammatory, its dual effect of calming the mind and reducing alertness can ease stress and elevate your mood at the same time. Sometimes, lemon balm is combined with valerian, a powerful herbal medicine for insomnia.

flower
allow her

pictured on pages 106–107

internal adornment and self-love

Sometimes, just surrounding yourself with beauty can have a profound impact on your sense of well-being. When I'm feeling down, I reach for simple solutions to change my perspective. When summer arrives, I add flowers to my water because a little adornment goes a long way. This recipe creates a moment of self-care and gives you permission to be indulgent—your wellness is worth the effort.

Sip this water all day, every day, as long as edible flowers are available. Once you drink your flower elixir, add the remaining flowers to your bath, providing yourself with some extra TLC.

makes 4 cups ||| takes 2 minutes ||| rests 2 to 12 hours ||| lasts 1 day in the refrigerator

ingredients

||| 4 cups water
||| 1 handful fresh edible flowers, such as angelica, borage, calendula, chamomile, honeysuckle, nasturtiums, pansies, rose, or squash blossoms

special tools

||| quart-size jar with airtight lid

1. Pour the water in a quart-size jar and add the flowers.
2. Seal the jar and let sit in a sunny spot for 2 hours, or in the refrigerator anywhere from 3 to 12 hours.
3. When ready to serve, pour the liquid into a glass, leaving the flowers in the jar.

edible flowers natural mood enhancers

Flowers can add antioxidants and vitamins A, C, and E to our water, along with the beautiful, mood-enhancing impact of color. Studies have shown that just being exposed to the color, shape, and fragrance of flowers can help elevate our well-being. Make sure your flowers haven't been treated with pesticides and are truly edible. Start with the suggestions above, then do some research on flowers you can find locally, or in specialty shops.

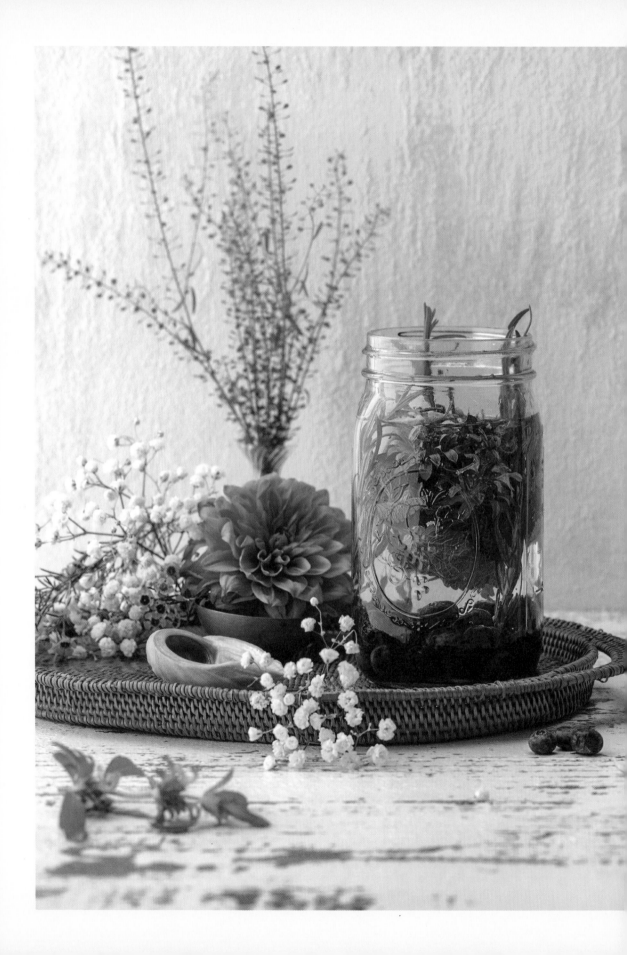

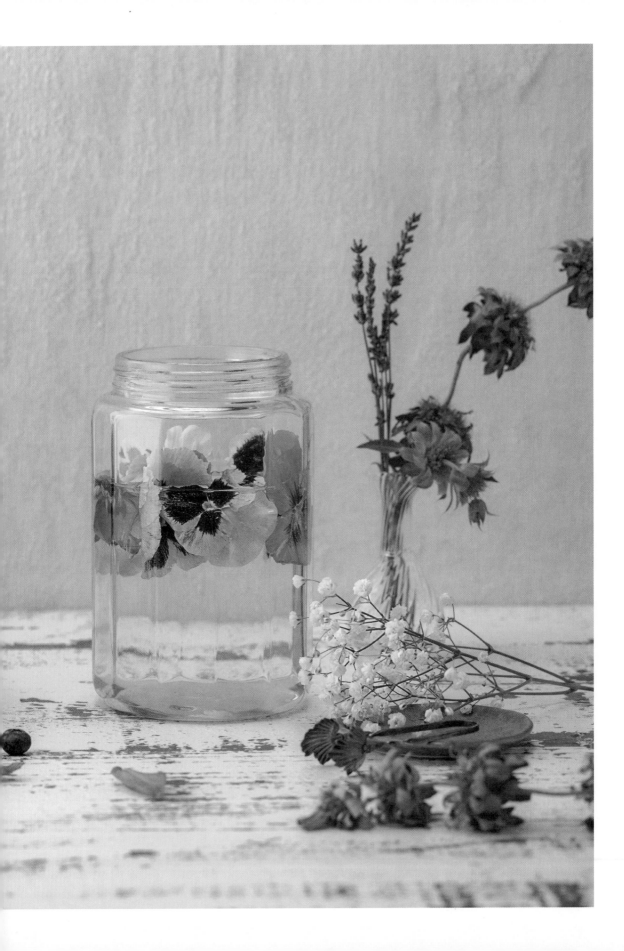

St.-John's-wort sunshine

alleviates winter blues

In the summer, I forage for St.-John's-wort and make tinctures, elixirs, and skin creams that help me overcome the challenges of long, dark winters. This recipe is created specifically for those who experience seasonal affective disorder. The addition of turmeric and ginger provides an added bonus of balancing the gut (the body's second brain).

An easy way to incorporate this joy-enhancing herb into your wellness regimen is to sip on this elixir daily. Make waking up that much easier by starting your day with a cup, and drink consistently for 6 weeks to experience the benefits.

Health tip: If you are taking pharmaceuticals, speak with your physician before adding St.-John's-wort to your rituals to avoid unwanted interactions.

makes 2 cups ||| takes 25 minutes ||| lasts 1 day in the refrigerator

ingredients

||| 1 cup water
||| 1 teaspoon dried St.-John's-wort
||| 1 star anise pod
||| ⅛ teaspoon ground turmeric or 1 (1-inch) piece turmeric root, sliced
||| 1 (1-inch) piece ginger root, sliced
||| 2 teaspoons maple syrup, plus more to taste
||| juice of ½ lemon
||| ⅓ cup fresh orange juice
||| 1 cup ice (optional)

special tools

||| French press
||| blender

1. Bring the water to a boil.
2. In a French press, combine the St.-John's-wort, star anise, turmeric, and ginger, and cover with the boiling water.
3. Let steep for 15 minutes, then press down the filter.
4. Pour the liquid into a blender, add the maple syrup, lemon juice, orange juice, and ice (if using), and blend for a few seconds, or until the ice is crushed.

St.-John's-wort northern sunshine

Grown in sunny northern climates, this plant thrives in less-than-optimal soil and produces bright yellow flowers. Many studies speak to the benefits of St.-John's-wort, including for treatment of mild depression and seasonal affective disorder. Some believe that it is a reuptake inhibitor of serotonin, dopamine, and noradrenaline, which are chemicals in the brain linked to depression and anxiety. It is also used for its antiviral and antibacterial properties in the treatment of herpes, shingles, and HIV.

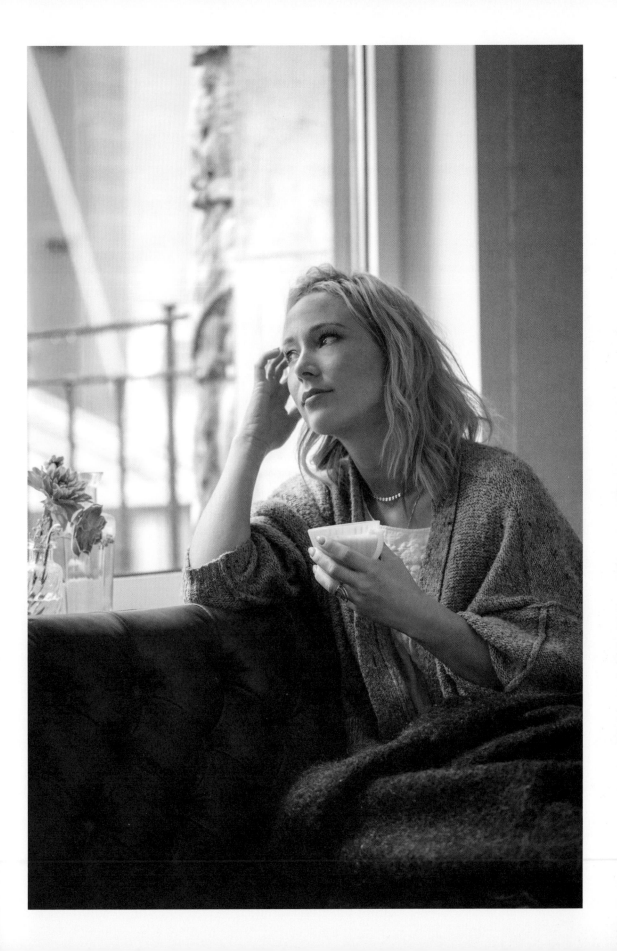

chapter ten

declare your devotion to your inner power and reclaim your sexual birthright

sexuality

embrace the pleasure

We are sexual beings with bodies that have been designed to experience pleasure. Fully engaging our senses with intention is a way to harness our sexual desires and access a feeling of completeness and power. Invest in your sensuality daily by expressing gratitude for your body and for your wholeness in every moment. Stoke your internal sexual fire with plants that have been fueling healthy, lasting sexuality and fertility for thousands of years. Each powerful in their own way, these elixirs will hydrate your body for optimal flow and allow the wisdom of ancient medicine to tone your body to give and receive.

Fo-Ti fountain of youth

aids feminine vitality

Feeling youthful and vibrant is at the heart of feeling sensual. When you support your inner vibrancy, you can keep the flame of youth alive while allowing your wisdom to shine through. This blood-building and longevity elixir will help you feel empowered, confident, and ready to embrace all life has to offer. With long-term use, Fo-Ti is known to help you express your energetic feminine powers, while reversing the onset of gray hair.

Take a moment, reflect on your inner radiance, and sip on this playful treat that tastes like a Creamsicle. Reach for this four to five times a week.

makes 1 cup ||| takes 5 minutes ||| best consumed immediately

ingredients

||| ⅓ cup fresh orange juice
||| ¼ teaspoon Fo-Ti powder
||| 1 teaspoon tahini
||| 1 teaspoon raw honey
||| ⅓ cup water
||| 1 handful ice

special tools

||| blender

1. In a blender, combine the orange juice, Fo-Ti, tahini, honey, and water, and blend until smooth.
2. Add the ice and blend again until the ice is finely crushed. Serve immediately.

Fo-Ti the qi increaser

A climbing plant also known as He Shou Wu, this rejuvenating herb is native to Southern China and is used to increase fertility in both men and women. Its most common use is premature aging prevention and it's thought to reverse hair loss and graying hair. Fo-Ti is also used as an overall wellness elixir to bring increased vitality to the body.

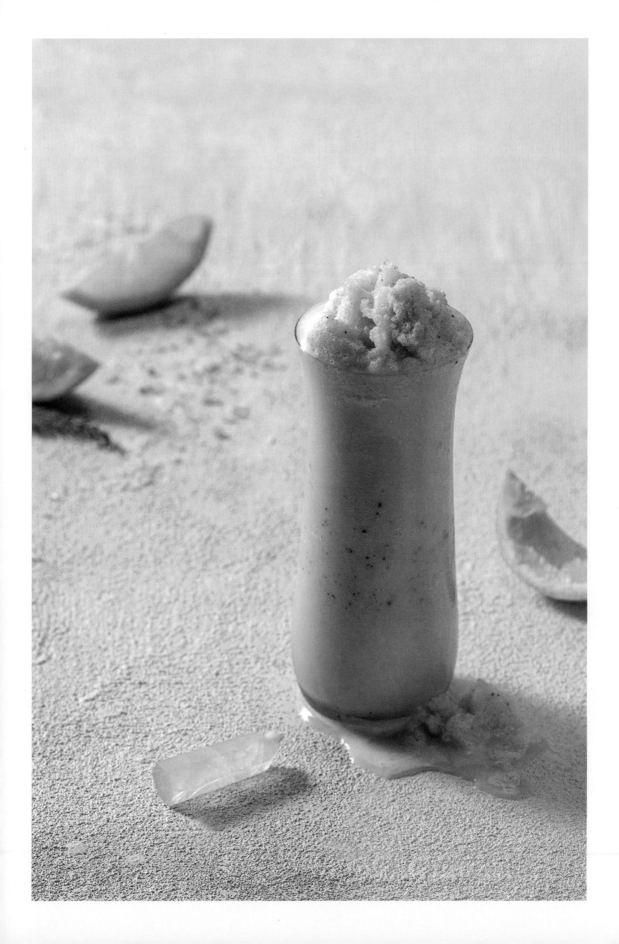

pine pollen pleaser

pictured on pages 116–117

aphrodisiac and hormone balancer

As I entered my thirties, I was searching for a boost to my sexual energy and found the answer in my own backyard—on a pine cone. If your libido is low and uncentered at times, this is often a result of unbalanced hormones. Pine pollen increases blood flow and energy, and balances hormone health. Support your internal chemistry to ignite sexual vibes and allow external chemistry to radiate with power and grace.

Sip this delicate, adaptogenic cocktail and get ready to share your radiance and self-love. Take two to three times a week as a foundational libido support, and before connecting with a love interest. Sprinkle rose petals on top for extra seduction.

Health tip: If you are on medication that prevents consuming grapefruit, substitute with orange juice.

makes 3 cups ||| takes 10 minutes ||| best consumed immediately

ingredients

||| 1 teaspoon dried Schisandra berries
||| 1 cup fresh grapefruit juice (from 1 large grapefruit)
||| 1 teaspoon pine pollen
||| 1 tablespoon coconut nectar or raw honey
||| 2 cups sparkling water
||| ½ cup ice, for serving (optional)

special tools

||| blender
||| quart-size jar with airtight lid

1. Soak the Schisandra berries in warm water until soft, then drain and set aside.
2. In a blender, combine the soaked berries, grapefruit juice, pine pollen, and coconut nectar, and blend well, until the berries are emulsified.
3. Pour the sparkling water into a quart-size jar, add the liquid from the blender, and mix gently to preserve carbonation.
4. Serve at room temperature or over ice.

note: For a special occasion, swap the sparkling water for sparkling wine.

pine pollen nature's hormone balancer

Pollen is produced by the male structures of a plant and creates sperm cells after a bee transports it to the female structures. Pine pollen is the only natural, plant-based source of the "wonder hormone" called DHEA, which is the precursor to male and female hormones. It aids bi-directional hormonal support, balancing both testosterone and estrogen in the body.

maca-
desiac

pictured on pages 116–117

enhances fertility

Fatigue is detrimental to our sexual flame, so fuel your fire with maca, a natural fertility supporter. Energy-boosting and fertility-enhancing properties will support those trying to conceive, and all those who feel like their drive has slowed down with the advancing years and lifestyle stressors.

Sip this in the afternoon, three to four times a week, during menopause, when attempting to conceive, or before an intimate encounter that deserves your full capacity. Serve it on ice, because you'll need to cool down after this drink.

makes 1 cup ||| takes 5 minutes ||| best consumed immediately

ingredients

||| ¾ cup Cinnamon Flow (page 89)
||| 1 tablespoon maca
||| ½ teaspoon vanilla extract
||| raw honey to taste
||| ½ teaspoon ashwagandha (optional)
||| 1 cup ice, for serving

special tools

||| blender

1. In a blender, combine the Cinnamon Flow, maca, vanilla, honey, and ashwagandha (if using), and blend until smooth.
2. Pour over ice to serve.

maca **nature's Viagra**

Sometimes called Peruvian ginseng, maca is in the same plant family as nutrient-dense favorites like broccoli and kale. Super nutritious, maca is also rich in beneficial plant sterols, chemicals that are related to the human hormones estrogen, testosterone, and progesterone, and are thought to mimic these hormones in the body. It is often used to increase sperm count and quality as well as libido in both men and women.

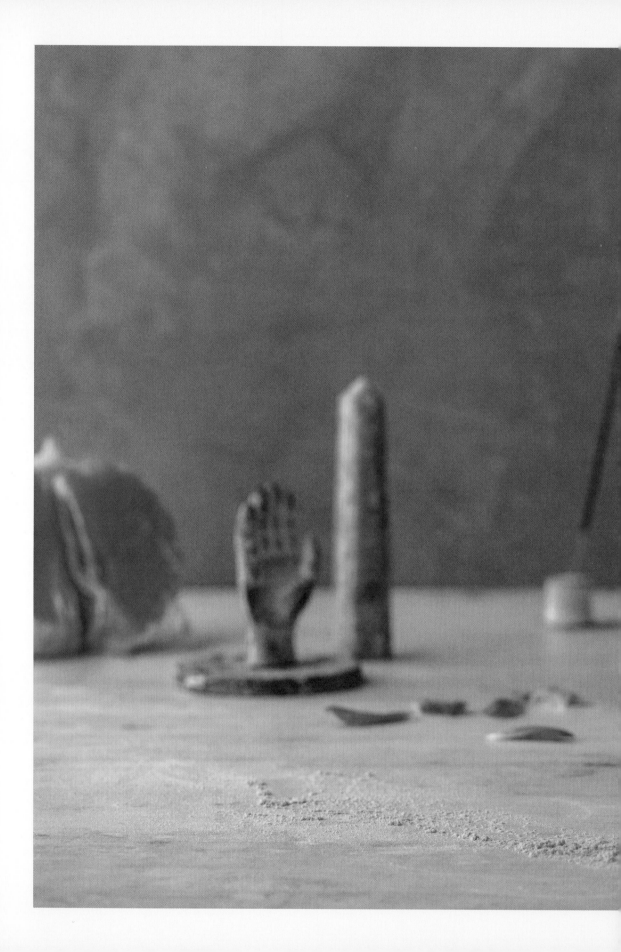

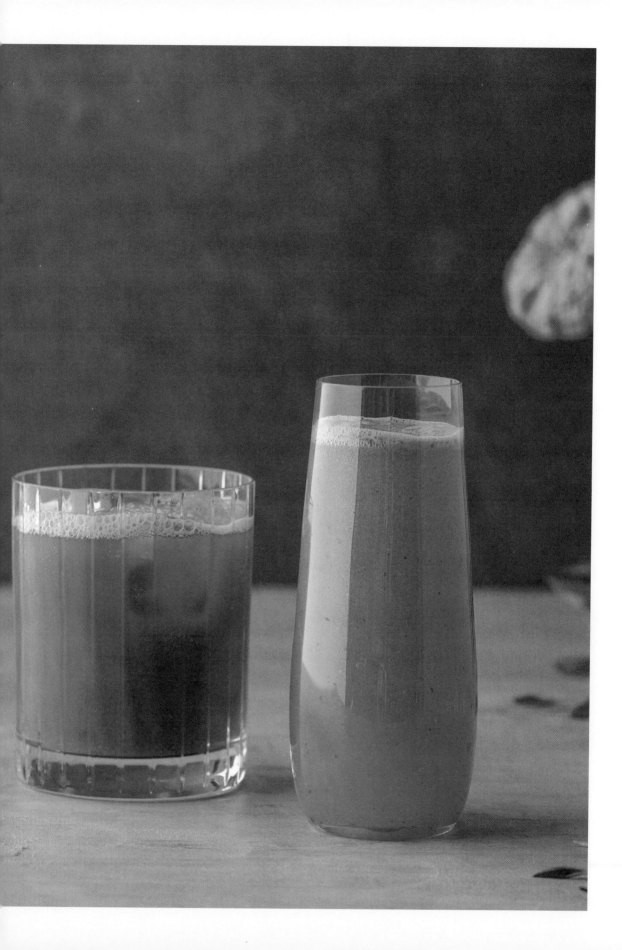

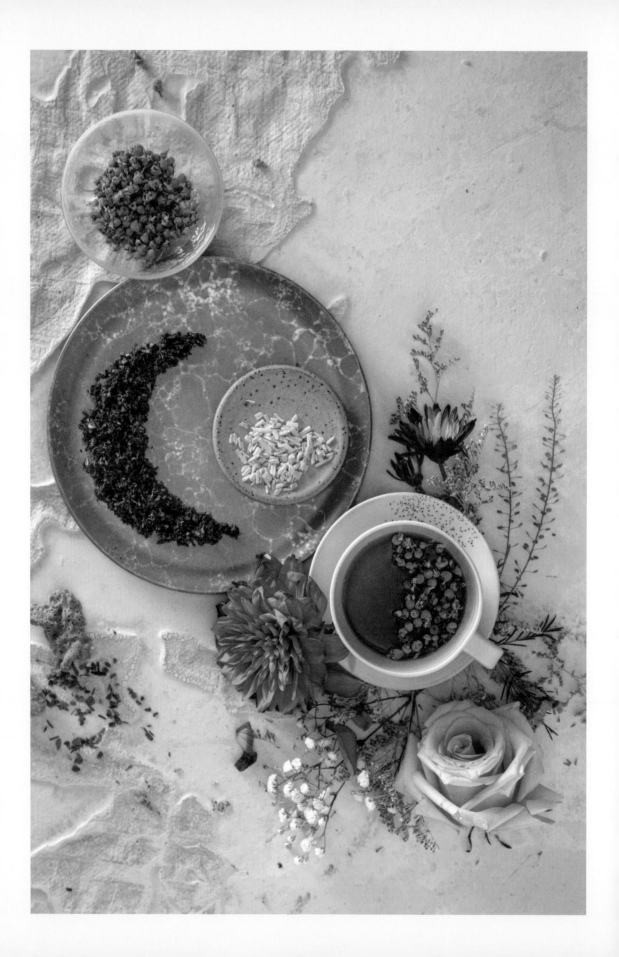

raspberry moon brew

empowers the female cycle

When I changed the script on my time of the month, I learned I could take pleasure in experiencing my body coming into alignment with natural forces. Nourishing our bodies with supportive elixirs creates a ritual of self-investment that we can look forward to during every cycle. Red raspberry leaf gently relieves menstrual cramping and nourishes the body.

Sip this elixir once a day, the week before and during your menstrual cycle, to manage symptoms and claim pride in your physiology.

makes 4 cups ||| takes 10 minutes ||| rests overnight ||| lasts 4 days in the refrigerator

ingredients

||| 4 cups water
||| 4 tablespoons dried raspberry leaf
||| 2 tablespoons dried chamomile
||| ½ teaspoon shatavari powder
||| ½ teaspoon ashwagandha powder (optional, for thyroid and hormone support)
||| 1 tablespoon Ceylon cinnamon chips

||| 1 (2-inch) piece ginger root
||| 1 teaspoon raw honey
||| juice of ½ lemon, plus more to taste

special tools

||| quart-size jar with airtight lid

1. Bring the water to a boil.
2. In a quart-size jar, combine the raspberry leaf, chamomile, shatavari, ashwagandha (if using), cinnamon, ginger, and honey, and cover with boiling water.
3. Seal the jar and store overnight in the refrigerator.
4. Using a strainer, strain out the solid ingredients, and return the liquid to the jar. Add the lemon juice before serving.

shatavari a woman with a thousand husbands

A member of the asparagus family, shatavari is traditionally used to increase circulation, hormone function, and to fortify the nervous system. It is often used to support women at all stages of their reproductive life, especially during menopause. In Ayurvedic tradition, shatavari is used to build *ojas*, or vigor, in the body.

chapter eleven

change the vibrations around
you and you will change the
vibrations within you

spirit

choose to connect

A simple, intentional act has the power to bring so much joy. Crystals harbor frequencies within their structure, and share those frequencies with our water when they're immersed in it, creating high-vibrational elixirs. And they are incredibly beautiful.

Use these recipes as a way to create a moment to focus on your intentions, and remember the commitment you made to yourself with every precious, energizing sip. Whether you're seeking clarity, happiness, or abundance, bring together the powers of water and minerals to transcend your current reality.

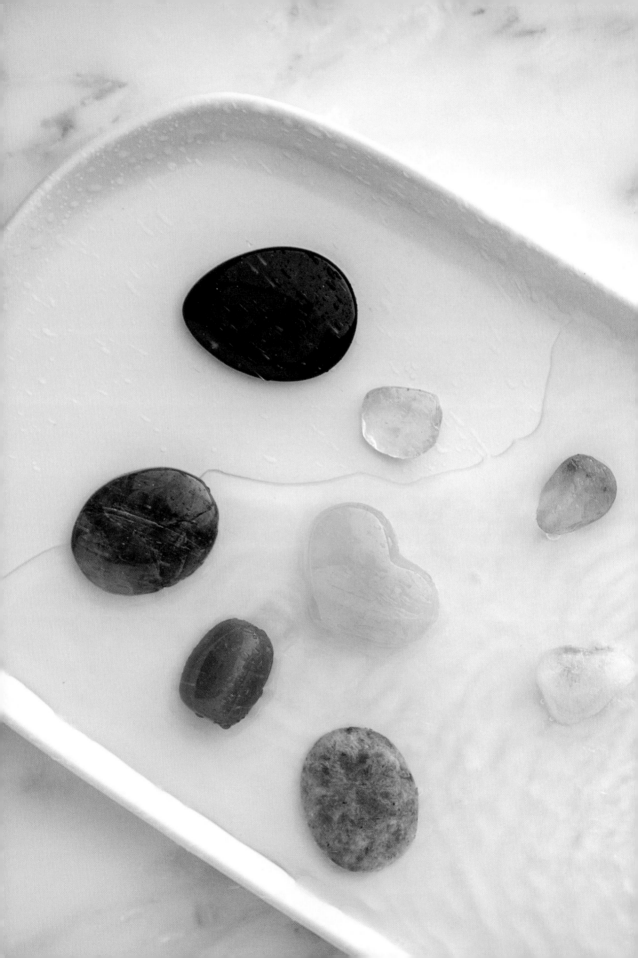

using crystals

Rocks and water have a beautiful relationship in the natural environment. When you bring these two elements together with intention, you are returning water to its natural home, side by side with the minerals that make up the earth. Re-energize your water after its journey through pipes and faucets, and reinvigorate it with the crystals and gems it knows. I encourage you to make this your own personal ritual, combining your favorite rocks and gems with your favorite mantras.

guidelines

||| Use only pre-tumbled crystals.

||| Some crystals are not safe in water because they may corrode, rust, or dissolve. Follow this simple rule of thumb: most crystals ending in *ite* are not safe in water, like calcite, lepidolite, malachite. Others are potentially harmful, like tiger's eye or selenite, which may contain asbestos.
Follow the recipes in this chapter for completely safe crystal water concoctions.

||| Unless you're making the crystal water in a water bottle with an infuser, pour your crystal water into a glass before drinking to avoid ingesting the crystals.

||| I like to recharge my crystals monthly. As crystals are susceptible to both positive and negative energies, they need to be restored to the positive by being cleared and recharged once in a while.
You'll be able to tell when your crystals need a recharge as the crystal water will lose its taste. When you need to re-energize your crystals, simply soak them in cool salt water. If possible, place them under a full moon and allow the lunar energy to help them do their best work.

preparing crystal water

1. Set an intention in your own words or use my guided intentions in each recipe.
2. Source your crystals and gather up a small handful.
3. Place the crystals in the bottom of a carafe or pitcher and cover with water.
4. Solar-soak the crystal water for 24 hours by placing it in a sunny spot like a windowsill. If solar-soaking isn't possible, place it in the refrigerator.
5. If desired, add specific fresh herbs or flowers to fortify your intention.
6. Drink pure crystal water within 10 days, and crystal water with herbs within 2 days. You can enjoy it as frequently as desired, keeping your intention in mind.

rose quartz and
rose water

self-love

I use this crystal to place my attention on forgiveness, detachment from old ideas, and the newness of caring deeply for myself and others.

intention

"I am worthy of giving and receiving real love."

makes 4 cups ||| takes 2 minutes ||| rests 24 hours ||| lasts 10 days in the refrigerator

ingredients

||| 1 handful rose quartz
||| 4 cups water
||| 1 tablespoon Bulgarian rose water

rose quartz the love attractor

This crystal is a pink specimen of the mineral quartz. It is abundant in areas of the world such as Brazil, Madagascar, and South Africa. Historically, rose quartz has been used to lower stress and address tension or dis-ease of the heart: heartache or heartbreak. Rose quartz encourages you to place your attention on attracting love and the newness of love and relationships, with yourself and others.

clear quartz and rosemary

clarity

When I feel like I need to access wisdom and clarity of thought, I make this elixir to help me focus and clear my mind.

intention

"I choose to walk in my power and to bravely
face obstacles with a clear mind."

makes 4 cups ||| takes 2 minutes ||| rests 24 hours ||| lasts 10 days in the refrigerator without the herbs and 2 days with the herbs

ingredients

||| 1 handful clear quartz
||| 4 cups water
||| 2 sprigs rosemary

clear quartz the master healer

A mineral composed of silicon and oxygen, quartz is the second most abundant mineral in the earth's continental crust. Historically, quartz is known as the Master Healer. It can amplify both thought and the effect of other crystals, absorb and store energy, and also regulate and release it. But it never stores negative energy.

citrine and flowers

abundance

I use this crystal when focusing on the potential and possibility of inviting rich, fulfilling relationships and experiences to enter my realm.

intention

"I am fulfilling my greatest potential and am able to welcome abundance in my life."

makes 4 cups ||| takes 2 minutes ||| rests 24 hours ||| lasts 10 days in the refrigerator without the flowers and 2 days with the flowers

ingredients

||| 1 handful citrine
||| 4 cups water
||| 1 handful fresh edible flowers, such as calendula, marigold, or rose

citrine the mentality of plenty

A translucent yellow variety of quartz, citrine ranges from pale to rich golden yellow, and gets its name from the French word *citron*, meaning lemon. Historically, citrine has been used as a stone to help manifest things in your life like prosperity, intuition, and personal power. As a quartz, it is a powerful amplifier, and is said to help soothe and ease fear or anxiety in association with the "lack mentality," or not believing that enough is available to you.

smoky quartz and lemon balm

empowerment

I use this crystal to harness the power of quartz, and remember to value living in the moment.

intention

"I am living my most powerful life, filled with joy and happiness."

makes 4 cups ||| takes 2 minutes ||| rests 24 hours ||| lasts 10 days in the refrigerator without the herbs and 2 days with the herbs

ingredients

||| 1 handful smoky quartz
||| 4 cups water
||| 1 handful fresh lemon balm

smoky quartz the advocate

Like other quartz varieties, this gray translucent quartz is a silicon dioxide crystal, found in regions of Brazil, Madagascar, and Mozambique. Historically, smoky quartz is associated with feelings of home and nature and is said to help ground you by promoting feelings of stability and security. It helps you live in your personal power and a more positive frame of mind.

obsidian and cilantro

detox

When I use this crystal, I am choosing to place my attention on the wondrous gifts of the earth, and to see true happiness in everything around me.

intention

"I choose to shield myself against negativity
and walk in truth."

makes 4 cups ||| takes 2 minutes ||| rests 24 hours ||| lasts 10 days in the refrigerator without the herbs and 2 days with the herbs

ingredients

||| 1 handful obsidian
||| 4 cups water
||| 1 handful fresh cilantro

obsidian the protector

A naturally-occurring volcanic glass, obsidian is created by quickly-cooled lava. Pure obsidian is found in many different places in the world, including Argentina, Australia, Iceland, and Japan. Historically, obsidian has been used to powerfully expel negative energies and to protect from the spiritual and psychic energy of others.

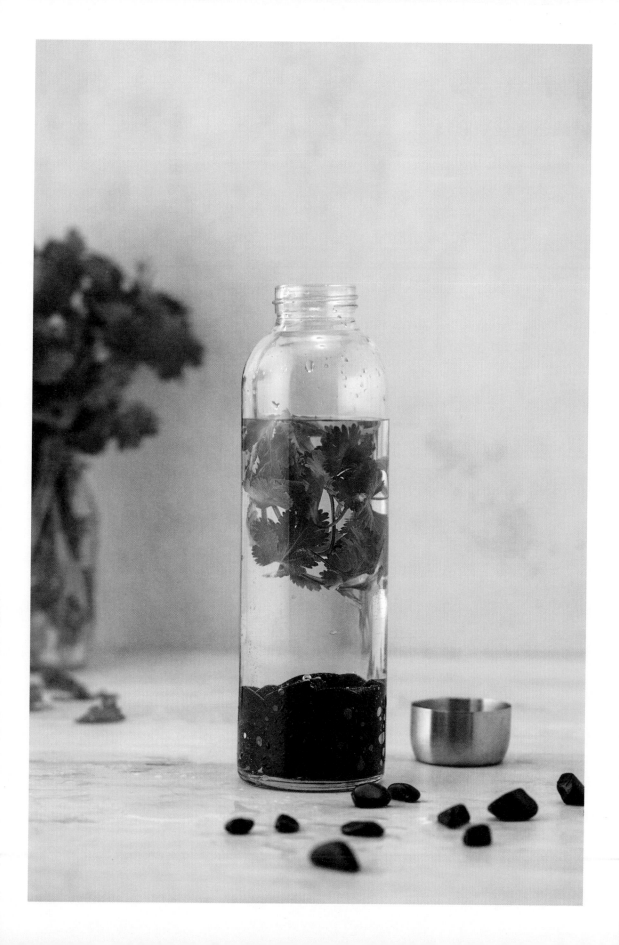

amethyst
and thyme

immunity

When I use this crystal, I tap into the powerful source of energy that allows our bodies to heal both physically and emotionally. I often have amethyst in my pocket.

intention

"I choose to live in a body that functions with
optimal health and limitless potential for wellness."

makes 4 cups ||| takes 2 minutes ||| rests 24 hours ||| lasts 10 days in the refrigerator without the herbs and 2 days with the herbs

ingredients

||| 1 handful amethyst
||| 4 cups water
||| 1 handful fresh thyme

amethyst   the positive guide

Some of the best and most vibrant varieties of amethyst, a rich violet-colored quartz, are found in Sri Lanka, Brazil, and Siberia. Historically, amethyst has been used to prevent intoxication—its name is derived from the Greek word *amethystos*, meaning "not intoxicated." Metaphysically, it is a natural stress reliever that can help the body function optimally, while ridding negative thoughts and energies that can weaken the immune system.

sunstone and lavender

happiness

When I feel I am surrounded by negative energy, I use this crystal to access spiritual protection.

intention

"I am light and happy. The universe sends me
gifts and I am filled with joy daily."

makes 4 cups ||| takes 2 minutes ||| rests 24 hours ||| lasts 10 days in the refrigerator without
the herbs and 2 days with the herbs

ingredients

||| 1 handful sunstone
||| 4 cups water
||| 1 handful fresh or 1 tablespoon dried lavender

sunstone   the light

Made of various minerals including red copper, sunstone is part of the feldspar family. It is commonly
found in Norway, Sweden, and the United States. Historically, sunstone carries the energy of the sun
god, Ra, which is the energy that brings all potential life to Earth. Quite literally, this stone is used to
infuse light and warmth, and to bless others with these positive energies.

ingredient shopping list and substitutions

item	find at	substitution
apple cider vinegar	grocery store	lemon or lime juice
ashwagandha bark or powder	health store, online	Siberian ginseng
astragalus bark	health store, online	reishi powder
basil (fresh)	grocery store	oregano, thyme (fresh)
beets	grocery store	–
blue-green algae (chlorella, spirulina)	health store, online	blue majik
blueberries	grocery store	seasonal berries
Bulgarian rose water	online	Moroccan rose water
burdock root	health store, online	milk thistle seeds
cacao powder	grocery store, online	–
calendula (dried)	health store, online	marigold (dried)
cayenne	grocery store	–
CBD oil	health store, online	–
Ceylon cinnamon bark or sticks	health store, online	–
chaga grounds or rocks	health store, online	–
Chamomile (dried)	grocery store, health store, online	–
cherries	grocery store	seasonal berries

item	find at	substitution
chia seeds (black)	grocery store	chia seeds (white)
cilantro (fresh)	grocery store	basil, parsley (fresh)
cloves	grocery store	–
coffee (ground)	grocery store	–
collagen (marine)	health store, online	–
cordyceps powder	health store, online	–
coriander seeds	grocery store	–
cucumber	grocery store	celery, watermelon
cumin seeds	grocery store	–
dandelion root	health store, online	burdock root
dates	grocery store	–
fennel seeds	grocery store	anise seeds
Fo-Ti powder (He Shou Wu)	health store, online	–
garlic	grocery store	–
ginger root	grocery store	–
ginkgo biloba (dried)	health store, online	gotu kola (dried)
gotu kola (dried)	health store, online	ginkgo biloba (dried)
grapefruit	grocery store	orange
green apple	grocery store	crab apple
Himalayan salt	grocery store, online	flaky sea salt
lavender (fresh and dried)	grocery store, market, online	–

item	find at	substitution
lemon	grocery store	lime
lemon balm (fresh)	grocery store	basil, mint (fresh)
lime	grocery store	lemon
lion's mane powder	health store, online	cordyceps powder
maca	health store, online	–
maple syrup	grocery store	raw honey
matcha	health store, online	green tea
MCT oil	health store, online	coconut oil
mint (fresh)	grocery store	basil, marjoram, rosemary (fresh)
moringa	health store, online	–
mugwort (dried)	health store, online	–
nettle (fresh or dried)	grocery store	–
orange	grocery store	grapefruit
pear	grocery store	–
peppermint (fresh)	grocery store	mint (fresh)
pine pollen	health store, online	–
raspberry leaf (dried)	health store, online	hibiscus (dried)
reishi powder	health store, online	cordyceps powder, ashwagandha powder
rhodiola powder	health store, online	–
rose petals (fresh or dried, food grade)	market, online	–

item	find at	substitution
rosemary (fresh)	grocery store	thyme, tarragon, other savory herbs (fresh)
royal jelly	health store, online	raw honey
sage (fresh)	grocery store	marjoram, rosemary, other savory herbs (fresh)
Schisandra berry (dried)	health store, online	hibiscus (dried)
sea buckthorn (fresh or dried)	health store, online	–
shilajit resin	health store, online	–
sparkling water	grocery store	soda water
St.-John's-wort (dried)	health store, online	–
strawberries	grocery store	seasonal berries
thyme (fresh)	grocery store	basil, marjoram, oregano, other savory herbs (fresh)
tocos powder	health store, online	–
triphala powder	health store, online	beleric myrobalan, black myrobalan, Indian gooseberry
tulsi (dried)	grocery store	basil (dried)
turmeric root	grocery store	–
valerian root	health store, online	–
vanilla bean	grocery store	vanilla extract
watermelon	grocery store	–

glossary

||| adaptogen

An herb that helps the body adapt and defend against internal and external stress factors by helping to balance and support the adrenal system. The name comes from its ability to "adapt" to what the body needs and support or restore normal functioning at any stage of wellness.

||| ashwagandha

This Ayurvedic herb is one of the most powerful adaptogens on Earth, balancing the adrenal system, regulating overall hormone levels, and supporting the body and mind through stressful times. It has many uses, including addressing anxiety, improving sleep, balancing blood-sugar levels, and boosting brain function.

||| astragalus

An herb that strengthens the lungs and qi energy while enhancing the immune system.

||| Ayurveda

One of the world's oldest healing systems, originally developed in India as part of Hindu culture more than 3,000 years ago. At its core is a belief in the idea of creating balance in bodily systems with diet, herbal treatment, and breathing techniques so that the body can heal itself. Like Yoga, it is considered a Vedic science, or a teaching that helps us reach our full human potential on a physical, mental, and spiritual level.

||| bioavailability

Rate at which nutrients are absorbed into your bloodstream. For example, you will absorb more collagen from a marine source than any other source.

||| blue-green algae

One of the original life forms on Earth, blue-green algae existed before any other plant life and can increase vitality in the human body. Consumed as a food and a medicine, it is incredibly dense with nutrients that are easily absorbed by our bodies. The benefits of taking blue-green algae are many, including protection against free radicals, support from bio-actives like plant sterols, and prevention of metabolic and inflammatory diseases.

||| botanical

A substance made from part of a plant, such as the bark, roots, or leaves, valued for its medicinal properties.

||| brew

An elixir made by bringing an herb in water to a boil, then simmering for a minimum of 10 minutes and up to 8 hours.

||| Bulgarian rose water

The most precious plant essence, gathered by steam distillation of fresh rose blossoms. Rose water is prized for its anti-inflammatory, skin-soothing, and beautifying qualities.

||| burdock root

A plant native to northern Asia and Europe that contains powerful antioxidants and helps remove toxins from the blood.

||| calendula

A flowering plant with anti-inflammatory and antibacterial properties, used to support soothing the skin from the inside out.

||| CBD oil

The cannabis plant contains more than 100 different chemical compounds known as cannabinoids, which interact with the body's endocannabinoid system. One of those cannabinoids is CBD, or cannabidiol (pronounced cann-a-bid-EYE-ol). CBD is non-psychoactive, which means it won't get you high—and there's a growing body of evidence around its numerous health benefits for stress, pain, focus, and memory.

||| chaga
An adaptogenic mushroom and one of the most potent antioxidants in the world. Chaga is used to support overall vitality and longevity.

||| chia
This superfood, native to Central America, comes from the same plant family as mint. Its high soluble fiber content creates the gelatinous substance you see when chia seeds are soaked. The fiber acts like a prebiotic and helps you feel fuller by absorbing fluid expanding in your digestive tract.

||| chlorophyll
Green plants harness the energy of the sun with chlorophyll, a pigment that absorbs light. Packed with powerful nutrients, minerals, and fatty acids, adding chlorophyll to your daily ritual creates an alkaline environment in the body, keeping body odor and inflammation at bay.

||| coconut nectar
A pure, raw sweetener with a low glycemic index. Safe for use by diabetics, or anyone wishing to maintain good health.

||| cordyceps
Alongside reishi, cordyceps is considered to be one of the most powerful adaptogenic mushrooms on the planet. Cordyceps can be used to create a powerful energy elixir, known to revitalize sex glands and the reproductive system. It also supports recovery from adrenal depletion and increases oxygen utilization.

||| cortisol
Sometimes called the "stress hormone," this steroid hormone is released from the adrenal glands in response to stressful situations. It regulates many processes, including metabolism and the immune response. When the body experiences ongoing stress, healthy cortisol levels are negatively affected.

||| dandelion
Often considered a weed, dandelion is taken as a diuretic to support lowered blood pressure, and also works as a prebiotic, encouraging positive gut flora. Early studies show that this antioxidant-rich plant can protect liver tissue when the body is under stress, or toxin levels are high.

||| Fo-Ti (He Shou Wu)
An herb known for rejuvenating qi energy, Fo-Ti encourages longevity and is used for calming the spirit and nourishing the heart.

||| German chamomile
A flowering herb used primarily to soothe digestive problems. It contains a naturally-occurring chemical compound called spiroether, which is a strong antispasmodic that eases tense muscles and intestines. This herb helps with indigestion, acidity, gastritis, bloating, colic, and irritable bowel syndrome. It is so gentle that it is suitable for children.

||| ginkgo biloba
An herb with circulatory, antiasthmatic, and anti-inflammatory properties, it is used to maintain plentiful blood flow to the central nervous system

||| gotu kola
An ancient herb, traditionally used in both Chinese medicine and Ayurvedic traditions to treat diseases related to the nervous system, and to improve memory and intelligence.

herb

A plant without a woody stem that is valued for its ability to produce medicine, aroma, or flavor.

herbal medicine

A system of healing and health that is founded on the use of plants and their extracts to treat disease and support optimal health and well-being. It is sometimes referred to as herbalism or botanical medicine.

hibiscus

High in vitamins C, this beautiful flower provides relief from high blood pressure and high cholesterol, as well as digestive, immune system, and inflammatory problems.

Himalayan salt

Mined from ancient seabeds and untainted by toxins, this variety of salt provides a rich source of more than 60 trace minerals used to detox and balance hormones.

lemon balm

A perennial herb from the mint family that has a mild lemon aroma. Often used in combination with other herbs, and to support anxiety, sleep problems, and restlessness.

licorice root

Helps the body process cortisol by stimulating the adrenal glands and mimicking the action of pharmaceutical corticosteroids.

lion's mane

A mushroom adaptogen used to support good brain health because of its special compounds that can stimulate the growth of brain cells.

maca

Sometimes called nature's Viagra, this plant from the brassica family is used to increase libido in men and women and has been used to help balance estrogen levels in women during menopause.

marine collagen

The most important structural protein in the body, collagen strengthens hair and nails, and is known to prevent joint pain and the formation of fine lines. Seek out marine (fish) collagen for the most bioavailable source of collagen for your body.

matcha

A finely-ground green tea powder of Japanese origin, packed with antioxidants called catechins, which have immune-boosting, cancer-fighting, blood pressure-reducing benefits.

MCT oil

A supplement containing good fats—medium-length chain triglycerides (or MCT). The triglycerides are broken down quickly by the liver and either stored as fat or turned into ketones for energy.

moringa

A tree so rich in health benefits that it is often called "the miracle tree." The leaves are rich in amino acids and highly bioavailable nutrients, minerals, and vitamins. A primary source of nourishment in many countries, moringa is celebrated for everything from increasing milk production in nursing mothers to restoring a damaged liver, which, in turn supports detoxification, fat metabolism, and access to nutrients.

mugwort

A plant used to boost energy and enhance lucid dreams. Taking mugwort is said to improve your dream recall and give you access to "divine" visions.

nervine

A medicine used to calm the nerves.

pine pollen

Collected from pine trees, and the only natural plant-based source of the hormone DHEA (dehydroepiandrosterone), pine pollen increases blood flow and energy, and brings vitality to male and female hormone health.

||| raspberry leaf
The plant source to the widely-eaten sweet berry. This gentle aid to relieving menstrual cramping and nourishing the body, is used in a uterine elixir in preparation for pregnancy and labor.

||| reishi
A mushroom and an essential adaptogen in Chinese medicine. Rich with the antioxidant beta glucan, reishi is one of the most powerful immune protecting substances available, boosting immunity, relieving stress, and promoting longevity.

||| rhodiola rosea
Similar to ginseng, rhodiola has been used for hundreds of years to enhance mental performance, and to promote physical and mental endurance. With anti-inflammatory and antidepressant qualities, rhodiola is best used for overcoming long-term stress and preventing burnout.

||| tulsi
Also known as holy basil, this variety of basil is an essential herb in the Hindu religion. Often used for its ability to relieve stress and keep the mind and body calm, it is also known to support positive digestion, relieving stress in the gut.

references

Ayurveda Palms. 2016. "Amazing Health Benefits of Hibiscus Tea." Medium, June 27, 2016. https://medium.com/@AyurvedaPalms/amazing-health-benefits-of-hibiscus-tea-33d5ea53c2d.

Britton, Jade. 2013. *The Herbal Healing Bible: Discover Traditional Herbal Remedies to Treat Everyday Ailments and Common Conditions the Natural Way*. London: Quantum Publishing Ltd.

Buhner, Stephen Harrod. 2012. *Herbal Antibiotics: Natural Alternatives for Treating Drug-Resistant Bacteria*. North Adams, MA: Storey Publishing.

Chevallier, Andrew. 2016. *Encyclopedia of Herbal Medicine*. New York: DK.

De la Forêt, Rosalee. 2017. *Alchemy of Herbs: Transform Everyday Ingredients into Foods & Remedies That Heal*. Hay House, Inc.

Empowered Sustenance. 2014. "How to Use Himalayan Salt." Empowered Sustenance, January 13, 2014. https://empoweredsustenance.com/himalayan-salt-benefits.

Gladstar, Rosemary. 2012. *Rosemary Gladstar's Medicinal Herbs: A Beginner's Guide*. North Adams, MA: Storey Publishing.

Godfrey, Anthony, and Paul Saunders. 2012. *Principles & Practices of Naturopathic Botanical Medicine: Volume 1 Botanical Medicine Monographs*. Toronto, ON: CCNM Press.

Higuera, Valencia. 2017. "Benefits of Shilajit." Healthline. https://www.healthline.com/health/shilajit.

Hutchens, Alma R. 1992. *A Handbook of Native American Herbs: The Pocket Guide to 125 Medicinal Plants and Their Uses*. Boulder, CO: Shambhala Publications.

John Douillard's LifeSpa. n.d. "Ashwagandha." LifeSpa. https://lifespa.com/ayurvedic-supplement-facts/ashwagandha.

Ku, Chai Siah, Yue Yang, et al. 2013. "Health Benefits of Blue-Green Algae: Prevention of Cardiovascular Disease and Nonalcoholic Fatty Liver Disease." *Journal of Medicinal Food* 16, no. 2 (Feb.): 103–111.

Murray, Michael T., and Joseph Pizzorno. 2012. *The Encyclopedia of Natural Medicine*. New York: Atria Books.

Noveille, Agatha. 2018. *The Complete Guide to Adaptogens: from Ashwagandha to Rhodiola, Medicinal Herbs That Transform and Heal*. Avon, MA: Adams Media.

Oliver, Kyra. 2017. "Sea Buckthorn Oil: The Ancient Greek Oil That Fights Major Diseases." Dr. Axe. https://draxe.com/sea-buckthorn-oil.

Project CBD. n.d. "The Endocannabinoid System." Project CBD. https://www.projectcbd.org/science/endocannabinoid-system/endocannabinoid-system.

St. Claire, Debra. 1997. *The Herbal Medicine Cabinet: Preparing Natural Remedies at Home*. Berkeley, CA: Celestial Arts.

WebMD. n.d. "Gotu Kola: Overview, Uses, Side Effects, Interactions, Dosing." WebMD. https://www.webmd.com/vitamins/ai/ingredientmono-753/gotu-kola.

Winston, David, and Steven Maimes. 2007.
Adaptogens: Herbs for Strength, Stamina, and Stress Relief. Rochester, VT: Healing Arts Press.

Yance, Donald R. 2013. *Adaptogens in Medical Herbalism: Elite Herbs and Natural Compounds for Mastering Stress, Aging, and Chronic Disease*. Rochester, VT: Healing Arts Press.

acknowledgments

Thank you to all those who hold the voices of the plants and their medicine. To the keepers of the earth, Ayurvedic doctors, Chinese medicine doctors, Indigenous peoples, herbalists, naturopaths, shamans, grandmothers, and to all healers around the world. Thank you for keeping these traditions alive to reach me and inspire the belief that plants are powerful and the human body is capable of more than we know.

I truly believe you are only as good as your team and no words can express how I feel about mine. Thank you for joining me on this crazy journey we call life.

I am grateful and humbled by the many serendipitous moments that allowed this book to be born.

Thank you, Chris Taylor and Michael Milstein for the introduction to Dovetail and your belief in my vision.

Thank you, Josh Williams and Mura Dominko from Dovetail, for allowing me the freedom to express my full creativity and for being such an amazing publisher. And thanks to the amazing prop stylist Sophie Leng and food stylist Elena Besser for creating magic on set.

This book would not have been possible without the talented Meghann Shantz. Your ability to gracefully share your craft and your innate knowledge has made working with you feel expansive, filled with flow, and definitely has raised the bar. I am looking forward to producing many books together.

Fiona Hepher, you are my right hand, my sister, my family, and I am honored to call you a friend. This book would not have been possible without you. Late nights, early mornings, and 48-hour sessions with a baby in your arms and a crazy timeline. We did it again and created magic. I am beyond inspired and grateful for what women are capable of thanks to you. Your ability to harness my vision and translate my words into my heart's meaning is matched like no other. You give new meaning to the phrase "dream team." When working with you, I believe anything is possible. Thank you from the bottom of my heart.

My team at PLNTSOP: Raj Teja, for encouraging me to think bigger, and Troy Felix, for supporting me through big leaps and helping me create the space to birth this book.

Chrystal Macleod, my mother of self-care, life organizer, and true inspiration for this work. I trust you to always be with me on this journey and know I'll always be with you on yours.

Brittany Gill, thank you for your photography contribution. I trust you to capture my most vulnerable moments.

Kristin Rondeau, thank you for applying your love and wisdom of the spiritual world to this book.

Rebecca Foster, thank you for helping me climb out of my creative block and supporting me through my lavender crisis. I am grateful for your talent and contribution to this book.

To Dr. Keith Condliffe, for sharing my healing journey with me over the last 12 years.

To Dr. Jenny Cundari, for your love of plant medicine and contribution to this book.

Kelly Deck, my soul sister. Thank you for providing your house for me to create this book, workshopping my bio, and cheering me on along the way. There are no words for my gratitude.

Nick Foster, my board of life director. Roy Yen, the president of my ethics. Jacqueline Jennings, my buffalo woman. Marika Richoz, my nourishment. Haitham El Khatib, for sharing your wife. Jenny McCrea and Laura Mooney, my roots. Cormac Norton, thank you for helping me start Nectar. Phil Webb, for your editing support. Dylan Gleeson, for staying the course with me over the years. I am grateful to you all.

Paul Gleeson, for rowing an ocean with me and setting me off on a life's course that has been beyond my wildest dreams.

Nico Schuermans, thank you for inspiring me to get off the grid, use my hands, and learn how to receive. You are a force of nature that I am grateful to share my life and days with.

To Caitlin Boorman, my right hand and cheerleader for years. Without you, this book would not exist. My team at Nectar, for sharing the juicy ride regardless of "juice life" moments. Your growth and belief in me have kept me on course. Thank you.

To my Dadaladdy, my foundation. Mom, my cheerleader. Clay, my everything. Emma, my sister. Layla, the love of my life.

Somewhere in this book, there is a little piece of all of you. Your wellness and joy are a huge inspiration for me and inspired me to create my elixirs. My heart is the fullest when I am nourishing you all.

index

Note: Page references in *italics* indicate photographs.

about the author

Tori Holmes is a nutritionist, a wellness entrepreneur, an author, and the co-founder of Nectar Juicery in Vancouver. In her early twenties, her spirit of adventure and her passion for life carried her through a grueling trip across the Atlantic in a 24-foot rowboat, as well as a very different but equally challenging adventure of facing a breast cancer diagnosis. Both experiences have made her turn to alternative medicine traditions from around the world, and she found her way back to wellness by utilizing the power of self-care beyond sick care. She is now a passionate advocate for the importance of water and hydration, alternative ingredients, and the power of our own bodies on the path to wellness. Today, she is a product developer and an ambassador for startup ventures in plant medicine.

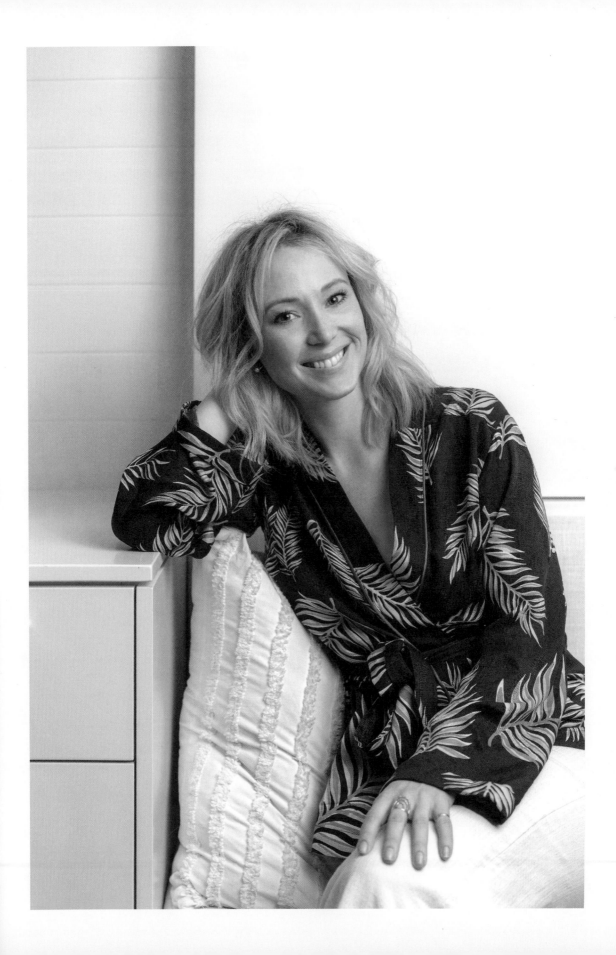